Joy of Pregnancy

Joy of Pregnancy

L C Gupta, M.D., D.Sc
Abhishek Gupta M.D. DRM

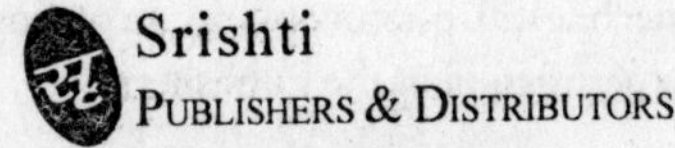

Srishti
Publishers & Distributors

SRISHTI PUBLISHERS & DISTRIBUTORS
64-A, Adhchini
Sri Aurobindo Marg
New Delhi 110 017
srishtipublishers@yahoo.com

First published by SRISHTI PUBLISHERS & DISTRIBUTORS in 2003

ISBN 81-88575-16-x

Typeset in AGaramond 11pt. by Skumar at Srishti

Dedicated

to

Dynamic, ideal couple

Jitender viz/Rama Viz

for their constant support

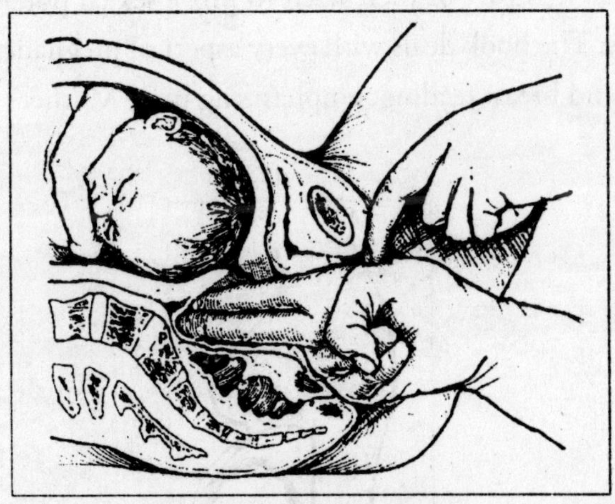

Diagonal Conjugate Measurement

PREFACE

Just after marriage it is natural for a couple to want to know each other and enjoy life for 2-3 years instead of becoming parents. Both men and women see contraception as a woman's responsibility, largely because it is the woman who is most affected by an unwanted pregnancy. Now many easy to use and reliable methods are available. One has to choose to meet his requirement.

Marriage is followed by pregnancy. Most of the women grow up thinking that child bearing is expected of them. Men also feel it is part of their need to prove sexual potency and virility. The book deals with every aspect of pregnancy, child birth and breast feeding, emphasizing that "Mother's milk is nectar".

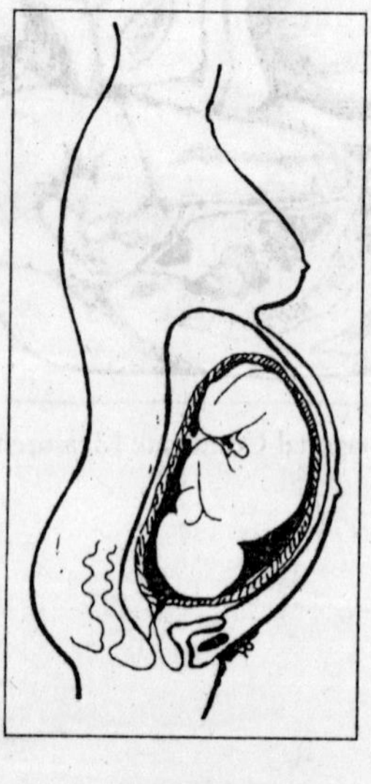

CONTENTS

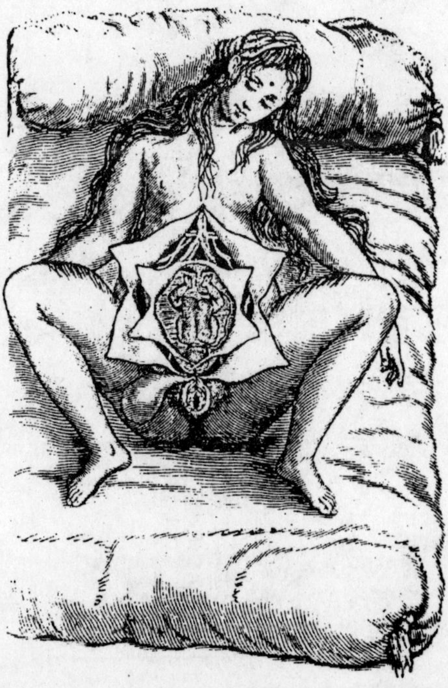

BIRTH PLANNING

What do you understand by birth control?

Birth control makes family planning possible by allowing the partners to choose the number of children and the length of time between births, which will be best for the health of the mother as well as that of her children. Birth control helps in making an intimate relationship more secure and more enjoyable by removing the fear of undesired pregnancy.

What is an ideal contraceptive?

- It should be reliable.
- It should be harmless and free from unpleasant side effects.
- It should be simple to use and cheap.

- It should allow for its effect to be stopped immediately.
- It should not interfere with intimacy.

What is a condom?

It is the only mechanical contraceptive used by man. It prevents the sperm from entering into the vagina during intercourse. By covering the penis it prevents the transmission of venereal infection. It reduces the sensation to glans penis and man may stay for a longer period. Condoms are easily available.

Is there any disadvantage of condom?

The disadvantage is that they can reduce the sensation and thus interfere with sexual pleasure of the partners. They also require an interruption of sexual activity as they have to be put on after erection but before introduction of penis in vagina. While taking it off proper care should be taken otherwise it may slip and the semen may spill over. Failure rate of condom is 2.5%.

Are female condom also available?

A prelubricated polyurethane condom for vaginal use are

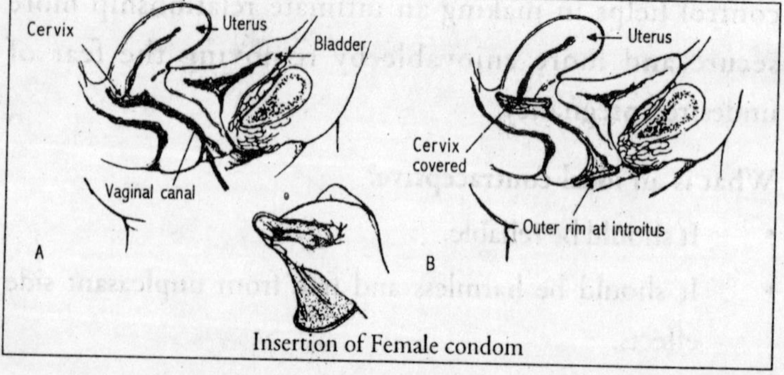

Insertion of Female condom

available. It has a closed end covering the cervix and an open end fitting into introitus.

What are oral contraceptives?

Pill has been the most common method of contraception and was first used about four decades ago. While condoms were used for centuries for contraception, I.U.D. was invented by Grafenberg in 1928. The idea of placing spermicides dates back to antiquity.

What is a combination pill?

It contains estrogens and progesterone. For a period of 21 days a dose of female hormones estrogen and progesterone is taken in the form of small tablets. It prevents releasing of an egg. Secondly daily low dose of hormones prevents the mucus membrane of uterus to get the ovum implanted.

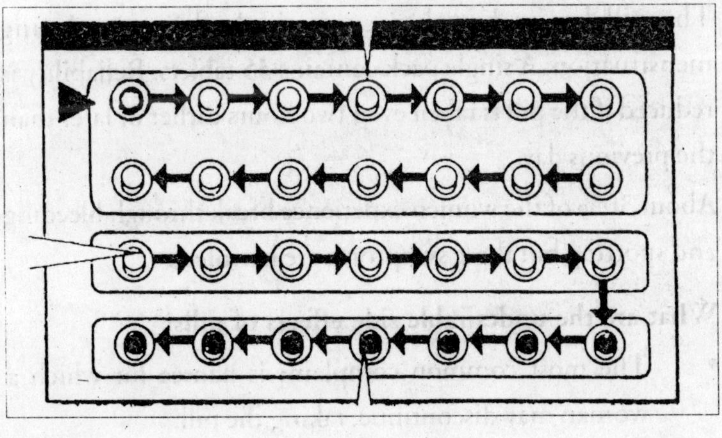

Pills

What is the effect of hormones over sperms?

Immediately after sex the sperm mass passes through the cervix and the uterine cavity into the fallopian tubes for fertilization. During the period of ovulation cervix becomes enlarged to facilitate the movement of sperm. Progesterone of pill impedes the ascent of the sperm.

Does a pill hamper the ripening of sperms?

One sperm can penetrate the outer membrane of the ova only after having undergone a certain ripening process. Progesterone hampers this ripening process.

Since pill interferes at every stage, it is highly reliable.

What are minipills?

With the mini pill the progesterones obstruct the ascent of sperm through the cervical canal and impede their ripening. Ovulation is usually not suppressed.

The pill has to be taken every single day even during menstruation. A single pack contains 35 tablets. Reliability is reduced if the pill is taken even two hours earlier or later than the previous day.

About 30% of the women experience break through bleeding and spotting but these symptoms are harmless.

What are the undesirable side effects of pills?

- The most common complaint is nausea for which a woman may discontinue, taking the pill.

- Bleeding, which occurs at times other than regular menstrual period is known as break through. This is due to the insufficient level of hormones in the body and will disappear when a pill with a higher dose is prescribed.

Will a woman on a pill gain weight?

The particular type of pill in use may influence the extent to which weight gain becomes a problem. Pills containing greater amount of estrogen will tend to cause the body to retain water. Lower estrogen level tablets will help.

What kind of skin reactions can develop?

Very young women may notice the appearance or increase of acne. There may be unusual hair growth and oily skin due to progesterone. A woman who is already having some skin problem should be more careful.

What are the side effects of pills?

Thromboembolism is a serious complication. Thrombus may be formed in the vein, resulting in pain and swelling of the distal part.

Certain women may complain of headache and also high blood pressure.

Are there any advantages of pills other than family planning?

Cramps caused by menstruation become less frequent. Unpleasant or even more irregular menstrual cycle may start with great accuracy. Painful breast tenderness is reduced.

Does the pill increase the libido?

Intake of pill may lead to a decline of sexual drive while its long term use may improve sexual relationship. It may be due to the elimination of fear of unwanted pregnancy. Fear of pregnancy always inhibits the ability to enjoy a relationship.

What to do if you forget to take the pill?

If you are on a combination pill it is not a serious matter because the reliability is not affected so long as the pill is taken within 36 hours.

As soon as you remember, take the tablet and continue as usual. At no cost should the pill be discontinued.

If you miss two pills, continue taking the pills but along with it a condom may be used every time for that cycle.

Can teenage girl take pills?

A young girl usually takes the pill as a means of birth control. Over this method they have control while the use of condom depends on the male partner. I.U.D. is often difficult to be used in a small uterine cavity.

Whatever may be said against the pill for this age group, it must be remembered that an undesired pregnancy or abortion could be a far greater evil for a girl still immature physically, intellectually and emotionally. Mini pills may not be taken by girls below 16 years because it hampers the growth.

What is intra uterine device?

The I.U.D. is a foreign body and this induces the white blood cells. These white cells make the sperm incapable of fertilizing an egg.

What is copper-T?

It is an intra-uterine device shaped in the form of the alphabet T and is moulded from polythylene. The device has a coil of fine copper wire wrapped around the vertical arm. Copper has antifertility capacity.

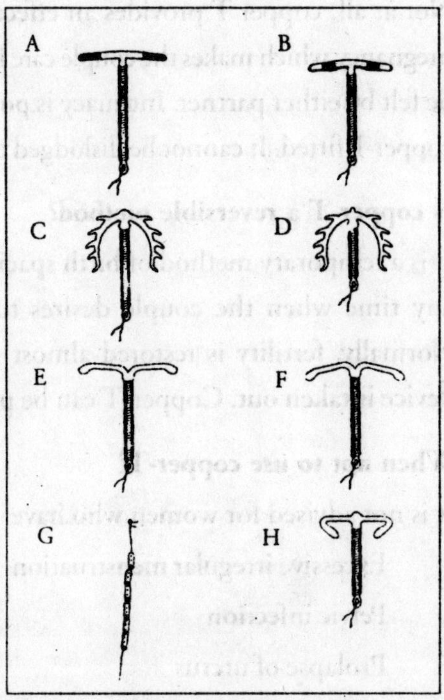

Different types of copper 'T'

How and when is I.U.D. implanted?

The procedure is simple but should be done by a physician or a trained nurse. I.U.D. is most easily inserted at the height of menstrual bleeding because the cervix is then open. There is very little chance of perforation for those who have already delivered.

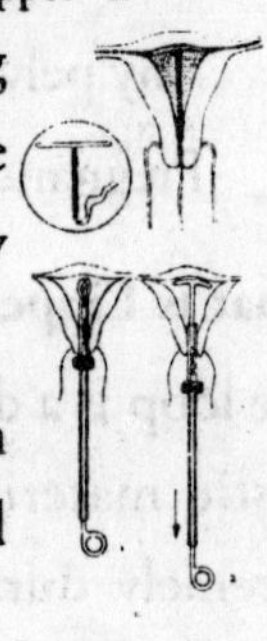

A. Copper-T

B. Insertion of copper -T

In breast-feeding mothers it can be inserted from the 6th week onwards. In case of MTP (medical termination of pregnancy) an I.U.D. may be inserted within 4-5 days of abortion or at the end of the first menstrual cycle.

Does copper T interfere with pleasure during sex?

Not at all, copper T provides an effective protection against pregnancy which makes the couple care free. Its presence cannot be felt by either partner. Intimacy is possible just after getting copper T fitted. It cannot be dislodged due to thrusts of coitus.

Is copper-T a reversible method?

It is a temporary method of birth spacing. It can be removed any time when the couple desires to have another child. Normally, fertility is restored almost immediately after the device is taken out. Copper-T can be placed for 5 years.

When not to use copper-T?

It is not advised for women who have

- Excessive irregular menstruation
- Pelvic infection
- Prolapse of uterus
- Retroverted fixed uterus
- Any pelvic bleeding
- Pregnancy

What is Lippe's loop?

The loop is a double 'S' shaped device made of polyethelane plastic material that is nontoxic, nontissue reactive and extremely durable. It contains a small amount of barium sulphate to make it visible on the X-Rays. The loop has threads made of fine nylon which project into the vagina. In India the loop is visible in 2 sizes i.e. 27.5 m.m. with a black tail and 30 m.m. with a yellow tail.

What is a safe period?

It is the time of menstrual cycle when ovulation is not expected for at least 5 days or has not occurred within 48 hours, so that the sperm and ovum may not get a chance to fertilize.

This method is suitable when menstrual cycle is regular i.e. of 28 days. Then ovulation would have occurred on the 14th day before the next period. The danger of fertility will then be from 9th to 16th day both inclusive. The rest of the cycle will be fairly safe. For extra safety it is always advisable to add another day on both sides.

What are the disadvantages of a safe period?

- Safe period intercourse means that marital relations are regulated by a calendar which to many people is annoying

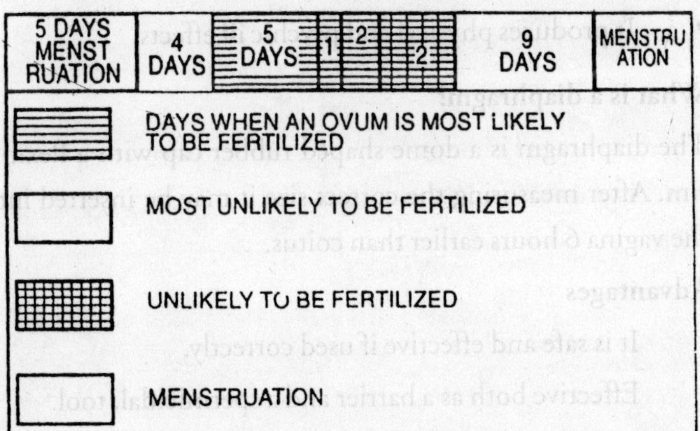

and frustrating if the couple is recently married or are serving in the army where leave is difficult to avail.

- On other days sexual intercourse may prove cold blooded instead of an expression of mutual love.

What is coitus interruptus?

It is an interrupted coitus. The man withdraws from the vagina before reaching climax and allows ejaculation to take place outside the vagina.

What are the disadvantages of coitus interruptus?

- There may be the failure of the male to withdraw in time. He may misjudge the moment of orgasm or else finds himself unable to control it. Sometimes delay in withdrawal may be due to the effort of the husband to allow his wife to reach a climax.
- The pre-orgasm urethral discharge may contain a few sperm cells to cause pregnancy.
- It produces physical and psychic ill effects.

What is a diaphragm?

The diaphragm is a dome shaped rubber cap with a flexible rim. After measuring the correct size it may be inserted into the vagina 6 hours earlier than coitus.

Advantages

- It is safe and effective if used correctly.
- Effective both as a barrier and a spermicidal, tool.

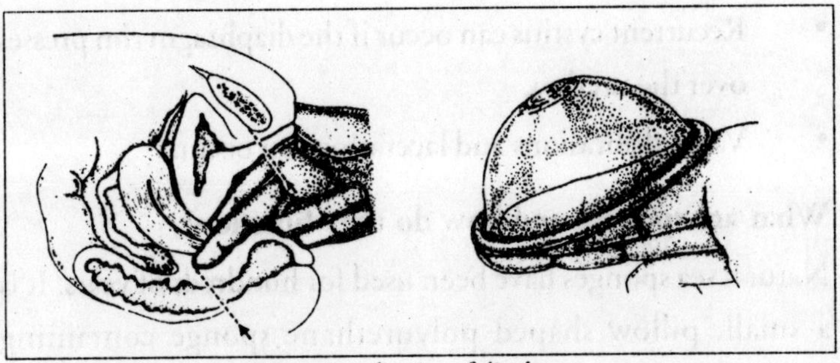

Measuring the size of diaphragm

- Interruption of sexual intercourse is avoided by early insertion.

Disadvantages

- Diaphragm is fairly large and conspicuous.
- It may be dislodged before or during intercourse.
- Inconsistent and incorrect use limits effectiveness.
- Must be washed and stored properly or deterioration of the rubber may take place.
- Requires fitting by a trained person.

Complications

- Allergic reactions to rubber or the spermicidal agent may occur.
- Foul smelling profuse vaginal discharge is produced when the diaphragm is left in place for too long.
- Monilial vaginitis can occur if diaphragm is not well cleaned and dried before re-use.

- Recurrent cystitis can occur if the diaphragm rim presses over the urethra.
- Vaginal abrasions and laceration can occur.

What are sponges and how do they function?

Natural sea sponges have been used for hundreds of years. It is a small, pillow shaped polyurethane sponge containing spermicide. It has a concave dimple on one side to fit over the cervix avoiding dislodgement during intercourse. The other side of the sponge incorporates a polyester loop to facilitate removal. It exerts its contraceptive effect by

- Providing a barrier between the sperm and the cervix.

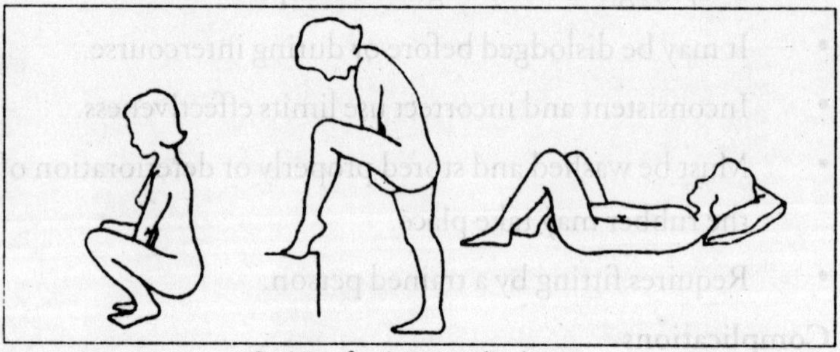

Position for inserting diaphragm

- Trapping the sperm.
- Releasing spermicide.

Advantages

- It is safe and effective if used consistently and correctly.
- It is easy to insert, soft and smaller than the diaphragm.
- Its use does not depend on the male.

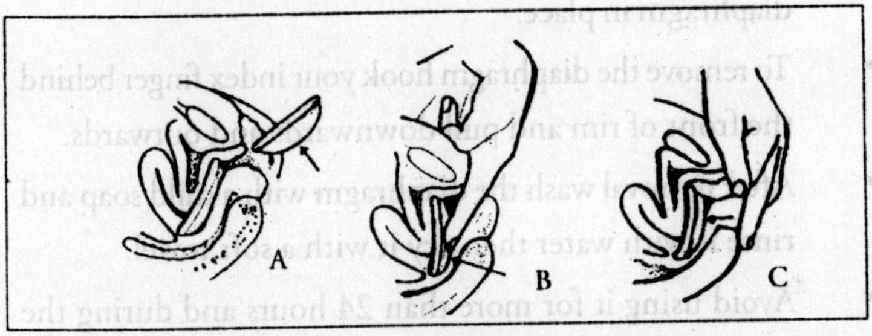

Application of diaphragm

- It acts as a barrier as well as a spermicide.
- May be left in place for up to 24 hours.
- It is not messy.
- It absorbs the semen so there is less discharge after intercourse.
- Single size fitting is not necessary.

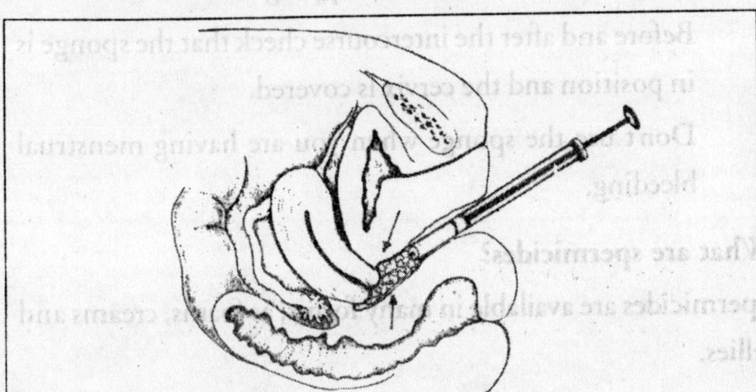

Insertion of jelly

- Put contraceptive jelly or cream into your diaphragm.
- Before inserting your diaphragm locate your cervix with your fingers. It feels like the tip of the nose.
- You can have a shower or bathe but don't douche with diaphragm in place.
- To remove the diaphragm hook your index finger behind the front of rim and pull downwards and outwards.
- After removal wash the diaphragm with a mild soap and rinse it with water then dry it with a soft towel.
- Avoid using it for more than 24 hours and during the menstrual cycle.

Important instructions for sponge users.

- Plan the insertion of sponge in soaked water before the intercourse. Dry sponge may not be effective.
- Wet the sponge with 2 table spoonsful of clean water, squeeze the sponge gently to remove excess water. It should feel moist but not dripping wet.
- Before and after the intercourse check that the sponge is in position and the cervix is covered.
- Don't use the sponge when you are having menstrual bleeding.

What are spermicides?

Spermicides are available in many forms, as foams, creams and jellies.

- Shake the container of foam atleast 20 times before you insert it.
- Try to insert a spermicide just before an intercourse. If you are using suppositories wait for 10-15 minutes so that it may dissolve before intercourse.
- If you are having intercourse more than once insert a spermicide before each act.

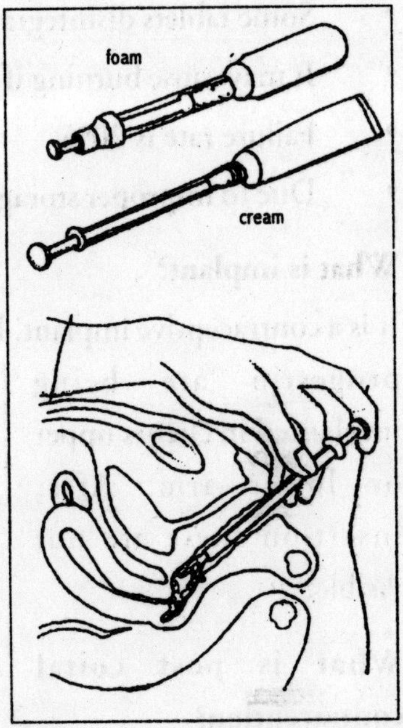

- If you want to douche wait for 8 hours after an intercourse.
- For better results use condom along with spermicides.

What are foam tablets?

When in contact with moisture the foam tablets generate foam. Each tablet is the size of a 25 paisa coin. One or two tablets after moistering are inserted deep into the vagina 5-10 minutes before sexual intercourse. The foam generated by tablets interferes with the movement of sperms. These tablets contain a spermicide known as penyl mercuric acetate or chloramin-T.

What are the disadvantages of foam tablets?

- Some tablets disintegrate when the vagina is dry.
- It may cause burning if there is cervicitis.
- Failure rate is 20%.
- Due to improper storage the tablets disintegrate soon.

What is implant?

It is a contraceptive implant. Its six tubes filled with synthetic progestin are being implanted in clients upper or lower arm. After insertion these are not visible.

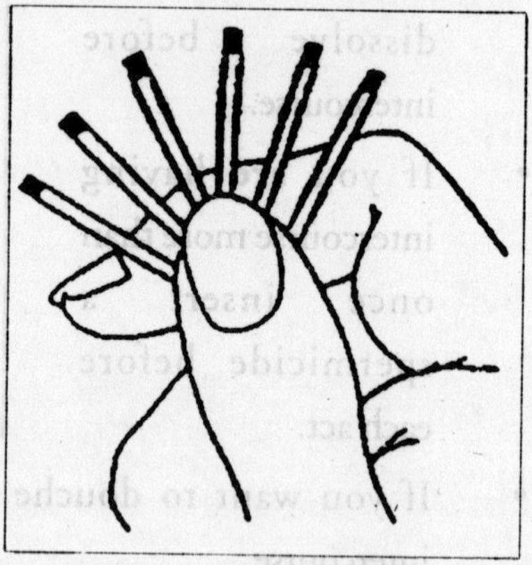

Contraceptive Implants

What is post coital contraception?

High dose of estrogen shortly following rape or unprotected intercourse will impede implantation or nidation of a possible fertilized egg. Once the egg is embedded in the uterine lining it will no longer be possible to induce it to move even with large doses of hormone.

Can I.U.D. help in post coital contraception?

The implantation of I.U.D. immediately following an unprotected intercourse can prevent pregnancy if the egg is

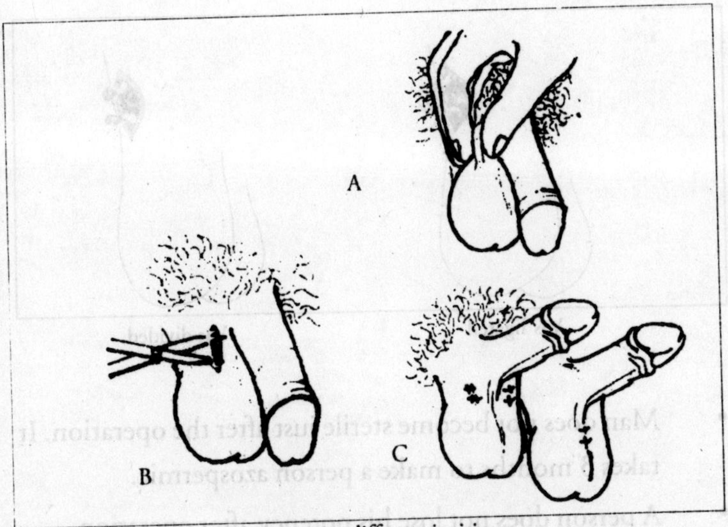

Vasectomy – different incisions

still mobile. It can be effective even up to 5 days following an intercourse. It may be left inside to serve against pregnancy.

What are the guidelines for sterilisation?

- The age of the husband should not be less than 25 years.
- The age of the wife should not be less than 20 years or more than 45 years.
- The motivated couple must preferably be having 2 living children and the youngest one more than 2 years.
- Consent of his/her spouse.

What precautions should be taken after vasectomy?

- Avoid intercourse for 15 days. Also use condom for 3 months till no sperm is found in 3 consecutive semen tests.

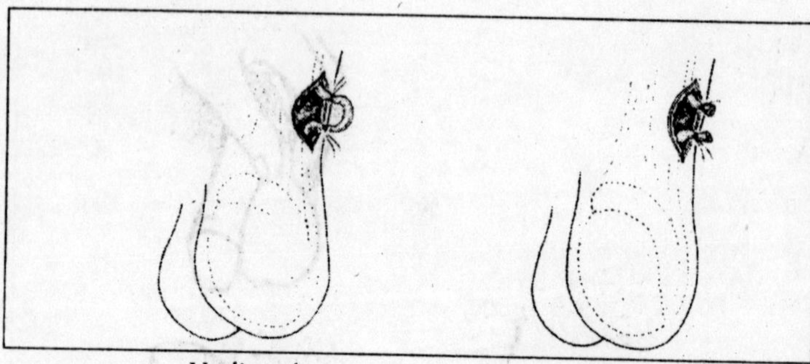
Vas ligated   Vas divided

- Man does not become sterile just after the operation. It takes 3 months to make a person azospermic.
- A person does not lose his potency after operation.

What is tubal sterilization for females?

There are about five operations which involve approaches either

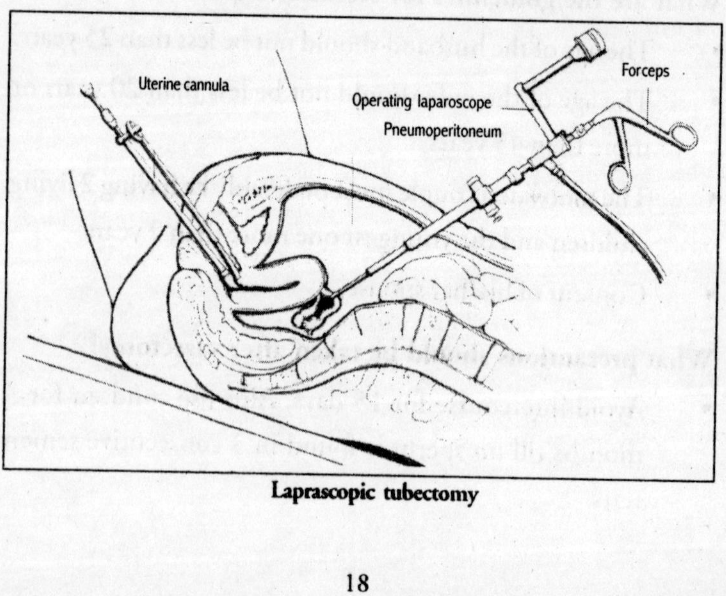

Laprascopic tubectomy

through the abdomen or vagina and tubes can be tied, clipped or sutured.

Most common and the least dangerous is the laproscopic sterilization with tubal ligation through abdominal wall. The procedure is very simple and the success rate is very high.

BEGINNING OF A NEW LIFE

How does human life begin?

A sperm cell fuses with the egg to initiate life. The moment a sperm and egg unite is the moment of conception. It takes place in the fallopian tubes. This fertilized cell migrates to the uterus.

Describe the sperm.

A sperm has a small structure. The head is only 1/250th of a

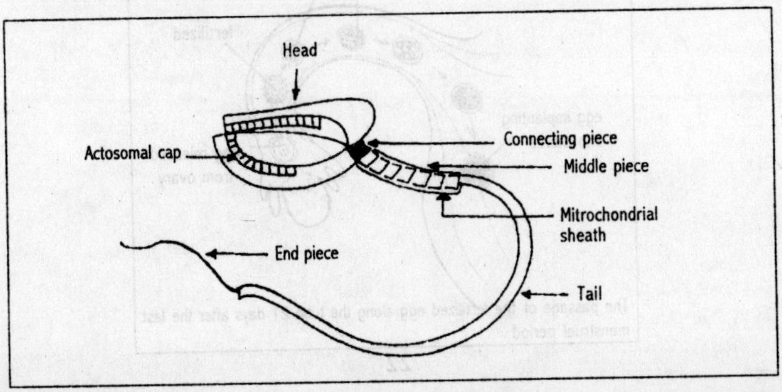

millimeter in diameter. The neck is short and cylindrical part containing mechanism for the movement of the tail. The tail propels the sperm with a speed of 6 m.m. in one minute.

Production of sperm is a continuous process. Then it reaches to epididymis where it may remain for several days. The sperms via vas deferens reach to sac like seminal vesicles and remain stored until ejaculation. The seminal vesicles together with the prostate secrete the seminal fluid.

What is an ovulation?

During each menstrual cycle about 250 ova commence to develop but only one is destined to be ripened and shed in the middle of the cycle. The fimbria helps to guide the fluid and ovum where fertilization takes place.

Life of an unfertilized ovum lasts about 12 hours and if it is not impregnated by the sperm it dies. Ovulation occurs on 14th day of 28 days cycle. So fertilisation has to take place on 14-15th day only.

What do you understand by fertilization?

The hyaluronidase of several sperms is required for liquefaction

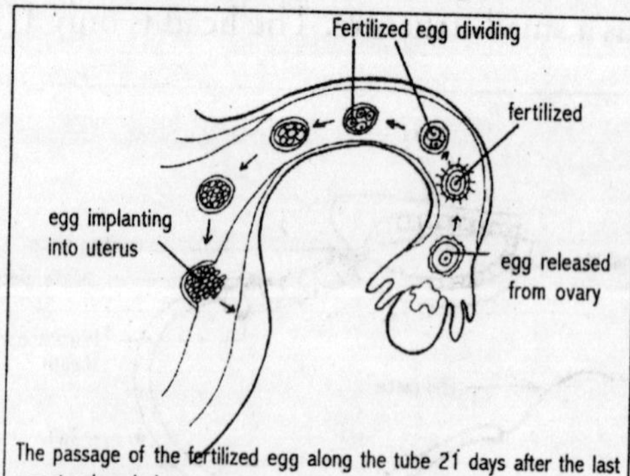

The passage of the fertilized egg along the tube 21 days after the last menstrual period

to allow one sperm to penetrate the egg. It is believed that the sperm makes head on contact with the ovum and penetrates the wall of the ovum due to its swimming velocity. During the first few hours the male and female nucleus will endow the offspring with its hereditary characteristics. Within a short time the nucleus divides into two, then four, eight, sixteen and so on.

What are multiple pregnancies?

It results in twins or triplets and is due to fertilization of one or two eggs shed from ovary.

(i) When one fertilized egg divides into two, it produces identical twins of same sex and same genetic make up.

(ii) If two eggs are released from ova at the same time and are fertilized by two sperms then two genetically different twins will develop. These are unidentical in shape and nature. Hereditary plays some part.

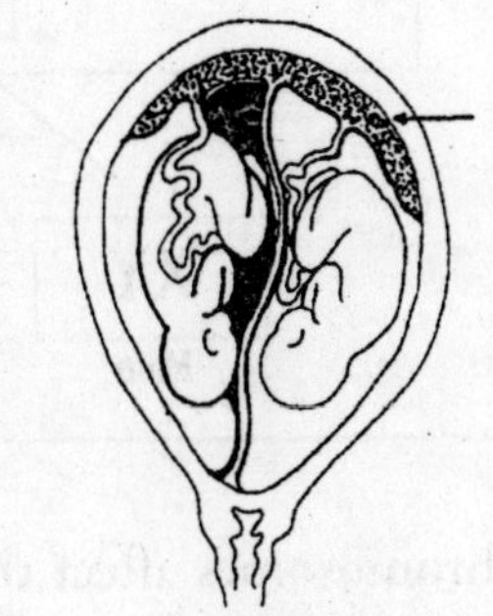

Identical Twins

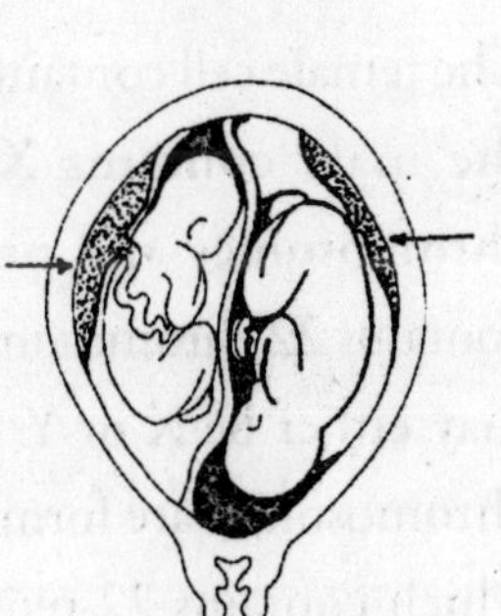

Non Identical Twins

How can the sex of the child be determined?

All human cells contain 44 chromosomes plus two sex chromosomes making it a total of 46 in all. The 44

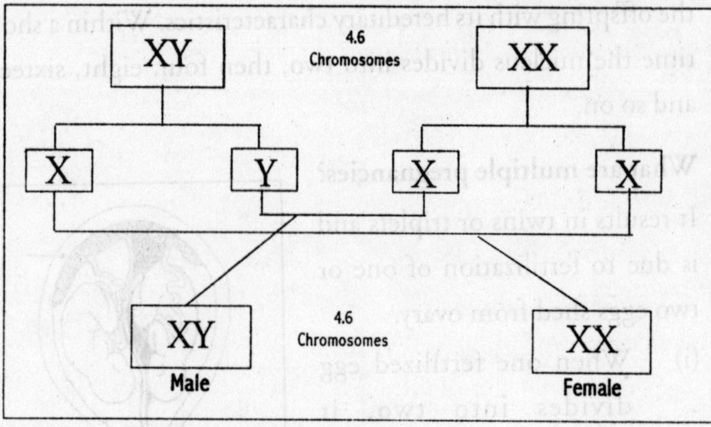

Sex determination

chromosomes affect the structure and function of the body and hereditary characteristics.

The female cell contains two sex chromosomes X and X while the male contains X and Y. The ovum consists of 22 chromosomes and one X chromosome while the sperm contains 22 chromosomes plus one of the chromosomes which may either be X or Y. Obviously equal number of X and Y chromosomes are formed. If the ovum is fertilised by a sperm which contains 22 plus X chromosomes, then the offspring will be 44 plus XX which is female. If the ovum is fertilised by a sperm containing 22 plus Y chromosomes the offspring will be male.

PREGNANCY

What are the symptoms of early pregnancy?

Failure of the menstrual cycle is the first sign of pregnancy. Although menses can also be stopped due to anemia, diabetes, tuberculosis or a sudden shock. Some women don't have any periods while using contraceptive pills. Sometimes there may be partially suppressed periods.

What do you understand by morning sickness?

Sensation of feeling sick may be felt as the first sign of pregnancy by some females. Nausea tends to be more severe in the morning hours. It follows an individual pattern, some may suffer it throughout the day for the first 3 months. There may or may not be vomiting. Ladies may not be able to tolerate the smell of cooking fat.

Early morning a piece of sweet and frequent small meal will help.

What is hyperemesis gravidorum?

Excessive vomiting known as hyperemesis gravidorum occurs occasionally and the woman usually is treated in a hospital. The vomiting does not harm either the woman or her child. Frequent sweetened drinks will help.

How is micturition affected?

There will be increase in the frequency of micturition. Majority of women pass urine between 4-6 times during the day and twice during the night hours. Frequency of urine becomes less marked during the fourth month.

Does taste also change during pregnancy?

Some women will recognise a strange taste in their mouth. Dislike for the cigarette smoke develops. Some like to eat mud, lime, pickles, sour mango etc. giving indication that they have become pregnant.

What kind of skin changes take place?

Dry skin may become still drier in early pregnancy. Some may develop dark spots on the face known as chloasma. It may persist even after delivery.

In later pregnancy white lines may be noted on distended abdomen.

What breast changes take place during pregnancy?

The premenstrual fullness of breasts continues. The breasts become full, slightly tender and more sensitive than usual especially in the area of areola and nipple. There may be a tingling

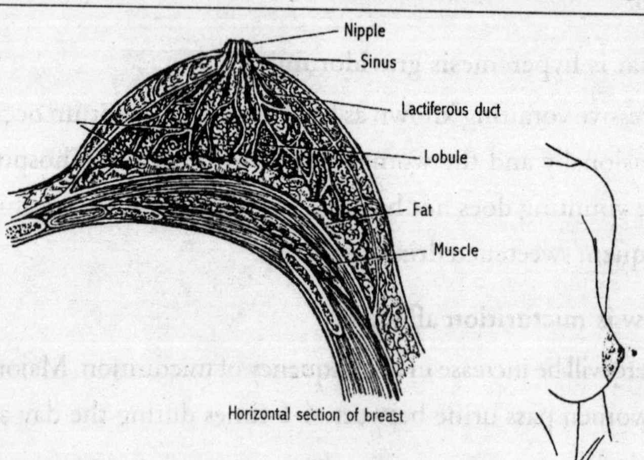

Horizontal section of breast

sensation. The nipple enlarges and becomes more prominent.

What do you understand by 'quickening'?

Feeling foetal movements in the first pregnancy starts between 18th-20th week.

What are common pregnancy tests?

Chorionic gonadotrophin can be detected in urine after the 35th day specially in the morning sample.

Now a days many reliable kits are available in the market and tests can be done at home too.

Ultrasound can also help you in detecting your pregnancy at the 6th week. Even fetal movements can be seen.

Can pregnancy be diagnosed clinically?

Internal examination will show bluish or violet discoloration of the vagina, softening of cervix, a slight enlargement and softening of uterus with palpable pulsation of uterine artery.

When should one go for the checks ups?

Your first prenatal clinic visit will be a long one because the doctor or the nurse will register you, fill up some forms. Your internal examination, blood and urine test will be done. Your blood pressure will be recorded. You may be

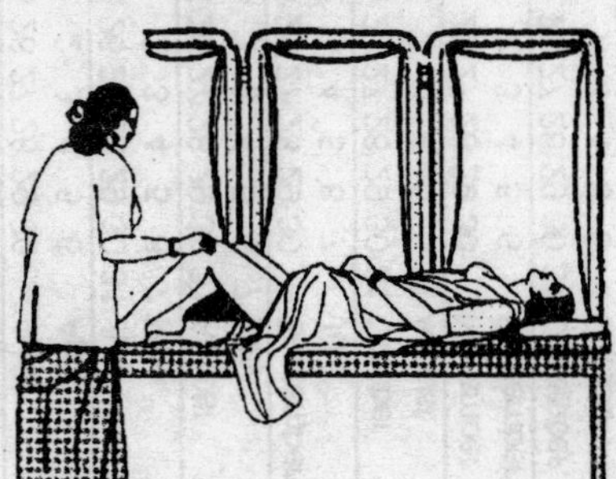

Estimating Your Baby's Date of Birth

January	1	2	3	4	5	6	7	8	9	10	11	12	13	14	15	16	17	18	19	20	21	22	23	24	25	26	27	28	29	30	31	Jaunary
October	8	9	10	11	12	13	14	15	16	17	18	19	20	21	22	23	24	25	26	27	28	29	30	31	1	2	3	4	5	6	7	November
February	1	2	3	4	5	6	7	8	9	10	11	12	13	14	15	16	17	18	19	20	21	22	23	24	25	26	27	28				February
November	8	9	10	11	12	13	14	15	16	17	18	19	20	21	22	23	24	25	26	27	28	29	30	1	2	3	4	5				December
March	1	2	3	4	5	6	7	8	9	10	11	12	13	14	15	16	17	18	19	20	21	22	23	24	25	26	27	28	29	30	31	March
December	6	7	8	9	10	11	12	13	14	15	16	17	18	19	20	21	22	23	24	25	26	27	28	29	30	31	1	2	3	4	5	Jaunary
April	1	2	3	4	5	6	7	8	9	10	11	12	13	14	15	16	17	18	19	20	21	22	23	24	25	26	27	28	29	30		April
January	6	7	8	9	10	11	12	13	14	15	16	17	18	19	20	21	22	23	24	25	26	27	28	29	30	31	1	2	3	4		February
May	1	2	3	4	5	6	7	8	9	10	11	12	13	14	15	16	17	18	19	20	21	22	23	24	25	26	27	28	29	30	31	May
February	5	6	7	8	9	10	11	12	13	14	15	16	17	18	19	20	21	22	23	24	25	26	27	28	1	2	3	4	5	6	7	March
June	1	2	3	4	5	6	7	8	9	10	11	12	13	14	15	16	17	18	19	20	21	22	23	24	25	26	27	28	29	30		June
March	8	9	10	11	12	13	14	15	16	17	18	19	20	21	22	23	24	25	26	27	28	29	30	31	1	2	3	4	5	6		April
July	1	2	3	4	5	6	7	8	9	10	11	12	13	14	15	16	17	18	19	20	21	22	23	24	25	26	27	28	29	30	31	July
April	7	8	9	10	11	12	13	14	15	16	17	18	19	20	21	22	23	24	25	26	27	28	29	30	1	2	3	4	5	6	7	May
August	1	2	3	4	5	6	7	8	9	10	11	12	13	14	15	16	17	18	19	20	21	22	23	24	25	26	27	28	29	30	31	August
May	8	9	10	11	12	13	14	15	16	17	18	19	20	21	22	23	24	25	26	27	28	29	30	31	1	2	3	4	5	6	7	May
September	1	2	3	4	5	6	7	8	9	10	11	12	13	14	15	16	17	18	19	20	21	22	23	24	25	26	27	28	29	30		September
June	8	9	10	11	12	13	14	15	16	17	18	19	20	21	22	23	24	25	26	27	28	29	30	1	2	3	4	5	6	7		July
October	1	2	3	4	5	6	7	8	9	10	11	12	13	14	15	16	17	18	19	20	21	22	23	24	25	26	27	28	29	30	31	October
July	8	9	10	11	12	13	14	15	16	17	18	19	20	21	22	23	24	25	26	27	28	29	30	31	1	2	3	4	5	6	7	August
November	1	2	3	4	5	6	7	8	9	10	11	12	13	14	15	16	17	18	19	20	21	22	23	24	25	26	27	28	29	30		November
August	8	9	10	11	12	13	14	15	16	17	18	19	20	21	22	23	24	25	26	27	28	29	30	31	1	2	3	4	5	6		September
December	1	2	3	4	5	6	7	8	9	10	11	12	13	14	15	16	17	18	19	20	21	22	23	24	25	26	27	28	29	30	31	December
September	7	8	9	10	11	12	13	14	15	16	17	18	19	20	21	22	23	24	25	26	27	28	29	30	1	2	3	4	5	6	7	October

booked for your delivery on the expected date of delivery.

How to calculate your expected date of delivery?

The average length of conception is 266 days.

Add seven days to the last menstrual period. Suppose your last menstrual period started on 10th Feb. add seven to it i.e. 17th Feb. and then minus 3 months. Then the due day of delivery will be 17th November.

Can you tell the sex of the unborn child?

Yes in the 16th week, with the help of ultrasound you can come to know the sex of the child but it is unethical to get the female child aborted.

How fundal height helps in knowing age of pregnancy?

Fetus is just palbable above the symphysis pubis by 12th week of pregnancy. It reaches to the umbilicus by 24th week. Uterine fundus grows 2 fingers by every 2 weeks. It reaches at xiphisternum by 36th week.

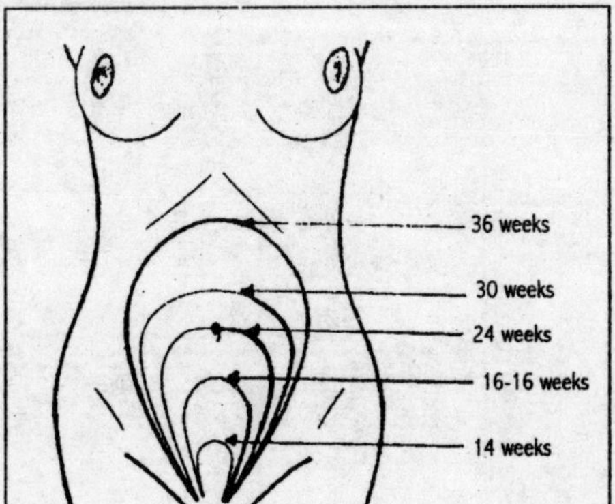

Fundal height

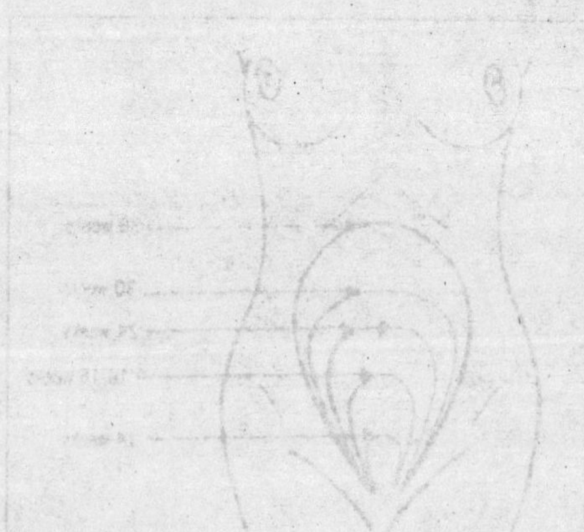

MISCARRIAGE

What is threatened abortion?

You develop some vaginal bleeding with or without abdominal pain. Your cervix is closed. Bed rest and sedatives will help you.

What do you understand by inevitable abortion?

It means your miscarriage has reached a point where it cannot be stopped. Bleeding becomes red and heavier. Passing of fetus and placenta will subside the abdominal pain.

What is an incomplete miscarriage?

Your pregnancy is terminated but you have eliminated only a portion of the foetus. It can result in infection.

While in a complete miscarriage the uterus expels all its

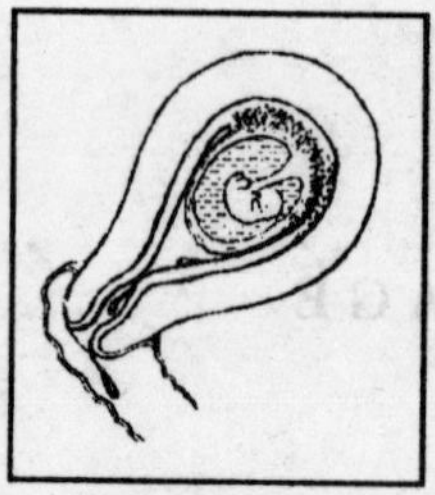

Threatened Abortion

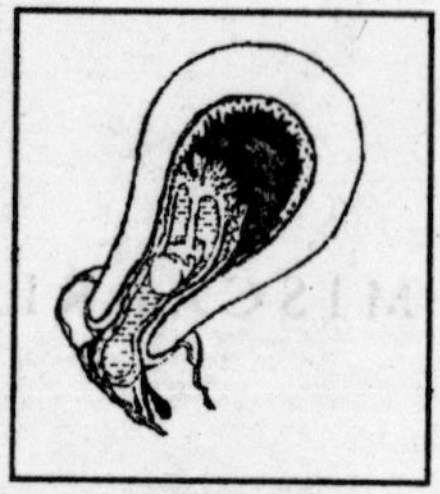

Inevitable Abortion

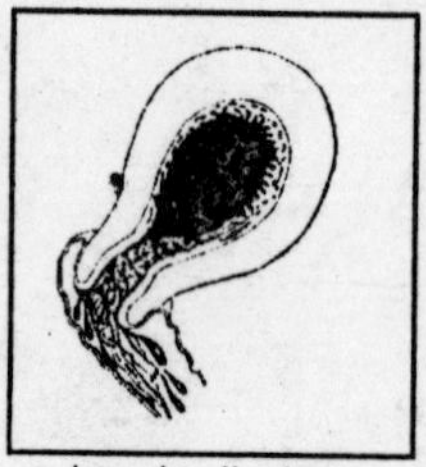

Incomplete Abortion

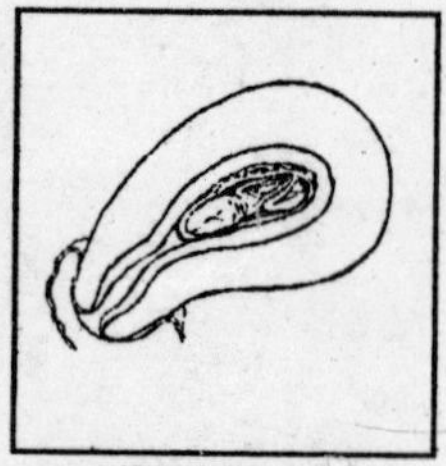

Missed Abortio

contents. You will continue to bleed for a week or so.

What is a missed carriage?

This means your fetus has died but the uterus has failed to expel it. Your uterus will fail to grow as it should. Dilatation and curettage operation will help you.

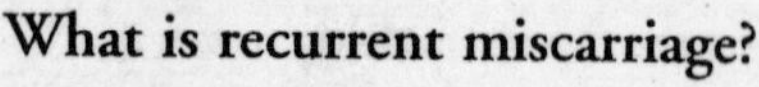

What is recurrent miscarriage?

There are very few women who miscarry each time one becomes pregnant. Hormonal treatment helps. One should consult an experienced doctor.

How do women cope with miscarriage?

Many will go under post natal depression. They develop the feeling of inadequacy, fear, guilt, sorrow and sometimes anger. You will require a sympathy of your husband and in-laws. But the best possible medicine for a miscarriage is to try again.

What do you understand by Rhesus sensitization?

The Rh factor can only give trouble when a Rhesus negative

woman is carrying a Rhesus positive child. After the first delivery a lot of Rh antibody will form a high concentration in her blood and a high concentration will pass into the fetus where it will cause massive destruction from anemia to heart failure.

A doctor should be consulted who will give proper vaccine.

What is phantom pregnancy?

It is also known as false pregnancy. A woman develops all the signs of pregnancy including loss of periods, nausea, sickness and breast changes and her abdominal girth begin to increase.

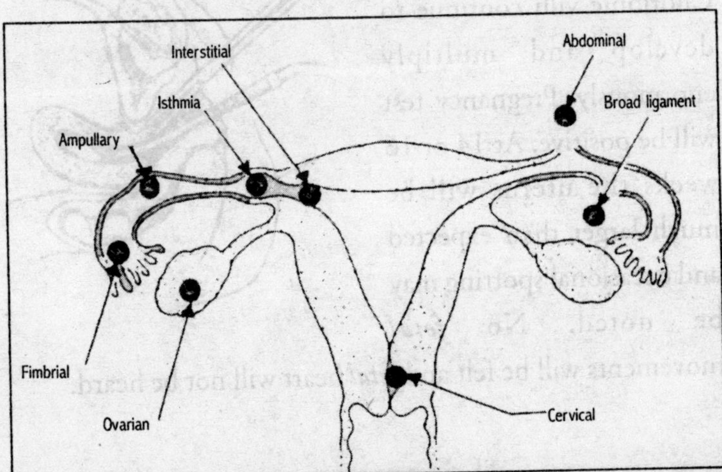

Sites of ectopic pregnancies

Women who develop a phantom pregnancy do so because they are very desperate to be pregnant. Careful psychiatric help is necessary.

What is an ectopic pregnancy?

Ectopic means simply 'out of place' is one that occurs outside the uterus. The likeliest site for such a pregnancy is the fallopian tube. The women will have all the signs and symptoms of pregnancy including a missed period but pregnancy cannot go to full term. The tube does complete the term successfully. A woman will complain of severe pain on the side and may show signs of collapse. There may be vaginal bleeding and surgical intervention may be required.

What do you understand by hydatidiform mole?

It is a strange abnormality of pregnancy in which only placental tissue develops. Chorionic villi continue to develop and multiply enormously. Pregnancy test will be positive. At 14 or 16 weeks the uterus will be much larger than expected and occasional spotting may be noted. No *fetal* movements will be felt and *fetal* heart will not be heard.

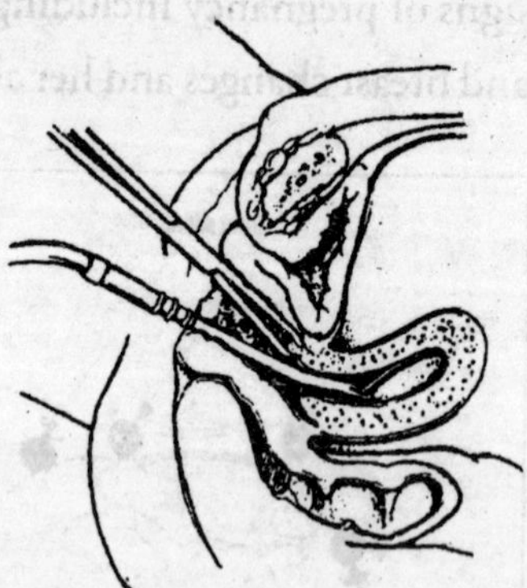

Hydatid form mole is to be removed by doing D & C.

What do you understand by placenta previa?

Placenta is normally situated in the upper part of the uterus and usually on the posterior wall. Due to a fault of implantation of ovum it is situated in the lower part of the uterus known as placenta previa. It will be below the head of the fetus and due to the pressure, separation of placenta always results in bleeding. Any bleeding after the 28th week should be reported to the doctor. In severe degrees of placenta previa caesarian section may be required.

What are the functions of amniotic fluid?

- Amniotic fluid helps in fetal movement.
- It provides a liquid environment of constant temperature.
- Its constituents vary to meet the requirement of constantly developing fetus.
- It provides a means of excretion of urine to the fetus.
- It functions as a shock absorber.

What is polyhyraminos?

The normal amount of amniotic fluid is one litre. If it is more than 2 litres there will be rapid enlargement of uterus and abdominal girth may enlarge from 15 to 30 cms. in a few days. Causes of chronic polyhydraminos include –

- Twin pregnancy
- Diabetes

- Pre eclampsia
- Congenital abnormalities of the *fetus*. It may lead to a premature labour.

Can there be fibroids with pregnancy?

Generally fibroids develop after the age of 40 and females become pregnant in thirties, still some may have fibroids.

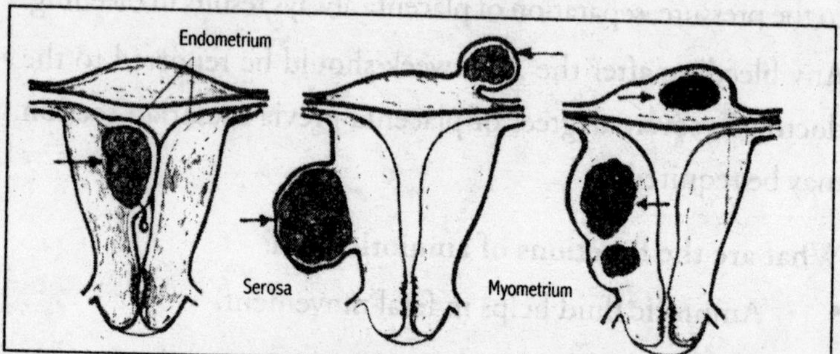

Submucous leoimyoma Subserous leiomyoma Intramural leiomyoma

Majority of fibroids have no significance and have no effect on a woman's fertility. Very large multiple fibroids may result in infertility and bleeding. Surgically these may be removed.

What do you understand by pre-eclampsia?

It is a condition in which two of the three classical symptoms are present.

- A rapid rise in blood pressure
- Protein in Urine
- Swelling of feet

There may be excessive weight gain also. Pre eclampsia very seldom occurs before the 20th week of pregnancy. Swelling of the face is nearly always part of the general gain in weight. All this can be detected in a prenatal clinic.

Eclampsia is a severe degree of disease. A female may have severe headache, visual disturbances, irritability and abdominal pain. Rest and medication is needed. Delivery is to be induced or caesarian section may be done.

How does placental insufficiency affect pregnancy?

Normal placenta is vital for a normal baby to be produced. Placenta reaches its full maturity at about the 34th week.

Complete failure of the placenta will result in an abortion. Occasionally placenta grows but fails to mature properly and will produce less hormone. The size of uterus will be smaller. Dysmature placenta provides a restricted supply of nutrition to the *fetus*. Hence it will develop slowly.

What happens on the death of foetus in the uterus?

If it occurs before the 28th week of pregnancy it will inevitably lead to a miscarriage. If it occurs after the 28th week it will result in delivery fairly soon.

If a woman feels her baby moves on an average ten times in a day, she need not to worry.

As soon as the baby dies the formation of progesterone and estrogen is dramatically reduced with resulting diminution of physical signs. The sensations of being pregnant disappear quickly. Breasts decrease in size. Swelling of the ankles disappears. Foetal heart will not be heard. After 3-4 days of the death the X-Ray of the skull will show an overlapping of skull bones. Ultrasound will be more accurate.

What is the body weight gain in pregnancy?

The gain in weight is due to many factors. There is an increase in the size of various organs specially breasts and the uterus. There is the weight of fetus itself with placenta and the amniotic fluid.

Weight of the baby	2.5 kg
Weight of the placenta	0.67 kg
Weight of the amniotic fluid	0.91 kg
Weight of the uterus	0.91 kg
Increase in the weight of breasts	0.67 kg
Increase in circulating blood volume	1.81 kg
Total	7.5 kg

Extra weight gain is due to fluid retention and fat deposit.

What happens in case of prolapse of the umbilical cord?

This is one of the emergencies where immediate delivery of child is to be done. In it the loop of cord protrudes below the head of the baby and appears in the vagina. If the membranes have ruptured they may be seen outside the vagina. During delivery if the cord is compressed, it could cause sudden death due to cutting of the supply of oxygen. So, if cervix is fully dilated then a forceps delivery could be done. If prolapse of the cord occurs earlier in labour then emergency caesarian section becomes necessary.

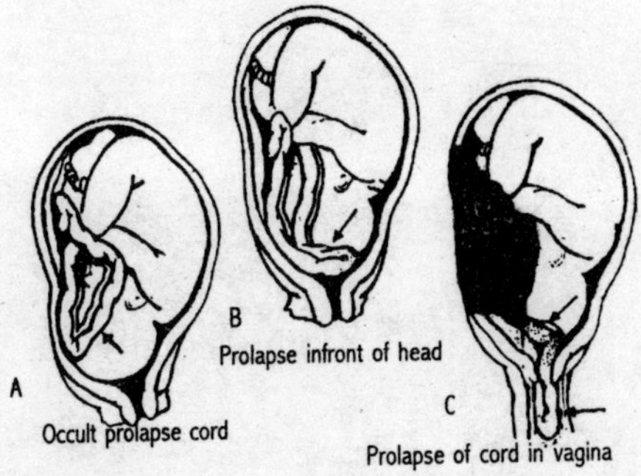

What is breech presentation?

About 3% babies present as breech i.e. buttocks present instead of fetal head. It is difficult to deliver such baby. Often genitals appear swollen and lumpy after a breech delivery.

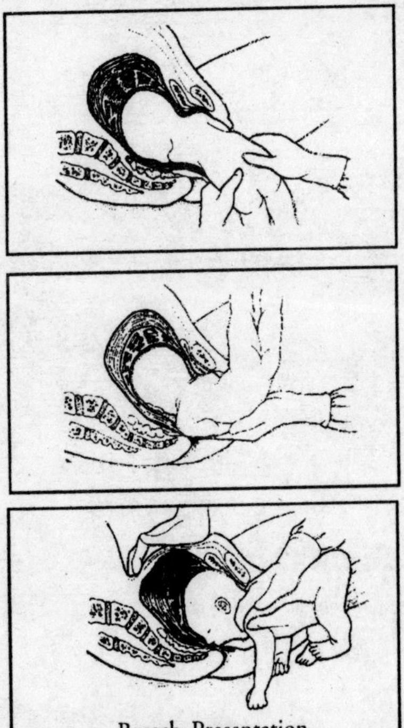

Breech Presentation

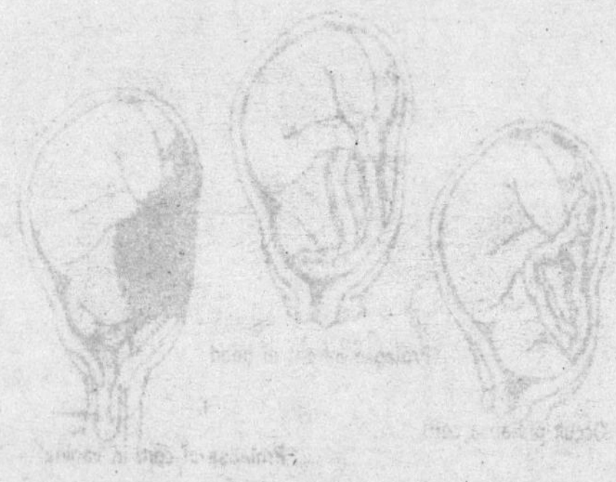

GROWTH OF THE EMBRYO

What is the growth pattern during 2nd to 6th weeks?

- 2nd week – The pregnancy consists of only one fertilised cell not visible to the naked eyes.
- 3rd week – The fertilized ovum travels along the fallopian tube and arrives in the uterus. In the end it embeds in the lining of the uterine cavity and is not seen by the naked eyes.
- 4th week – At the end eyes may be located.
- 5th week – Pregnancy is 2 m.m. in length. The spine is beginning to form.
- 6th week – The formation of head, chest and abdominal cavity starts. The spinal cord is formed. The heart is forming. Heart movements can be seen.

What develops in the 7th and 8th week?

- 7th week – The arms and legs are easily seen. The heart has started beating regularly. Liver and kidneys have developed. Eyes and ears start forming. The nose is not yet formed.
- 8th week – All the major internal organs are formed. The lungs have grown. The head of the fetus is still very large. The face is assuming some recognisable features. The limbs continue to enlarge.

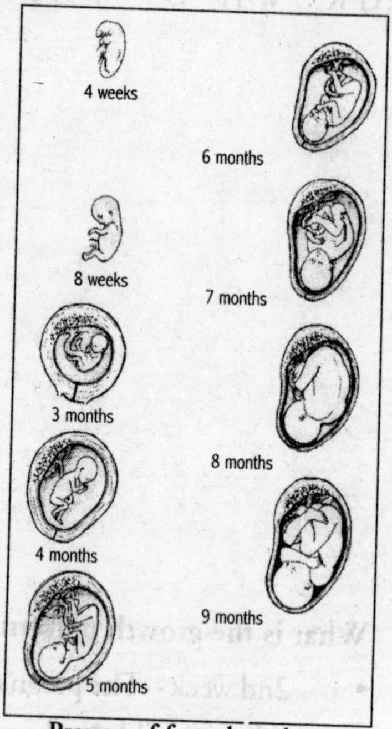

Progress of fetus throughout pregnancy

What shape does the fetus take during 9th to 12 the weeks?

- 9th week – It develops a mature appearance. The head is still bent towards the chest. The development of the eyes is complete. The nose has appeared. The limbs continue to grow. The movements are definite. Length is 3 cms and the weight is 2 grams.
- 10th week – Eyes have grown considerably. The inner part of the ear is complete. The face is more recognisable.

Ankles and wrists have formed. The umbilical cord is properly formed. The fetus now is 4.5 cm and its weight is 5 grams.

- 11th week – The fetus is easily recognised as a small human being. The head continues to grow in round shape and the face is developing fast. The eyes are completely formed. The movement of limbs and spine increases. The ovaries or testicles have formed. The length of fetus is 5.5 cm and weight is 10 grams.
- 12th week – The face is properly formed and eyelids are also present. Muscular development in the body and limbs increases. The growth of external genitals continues. Length of the embryo is 6.5 cms and weight is about 18 grams.

How does the fetus look during 13 to 24 weeks of pregnancy?

- 13th week – The uterus is distended. It contains 100 ml of amniotic fluid. The head is rounded. The face is formed with mouth, nose and eyes properly developed. Internal organs are also formed. Lungs, liver, kidney continue to grow. Subcutaneous fat is laid down. The length is about 7.5 cms and weighs about 30 grams.
- 16th week – Limbs are properly formed. Finger and toes are normal and nails are present. Sex of fetus is now obvious. A fine downy hair, lanugo forms over the whole fetus. Length of the baby is 16 cm and weighs about 135 gm.

- 20th week – The baby is growing rapidly in length and weight. Hair appears on the head. Muscle is rapidly increasing and active movements can be felt by the mother. Length is 25.5 cms and it weighs 340 gram.

How is the development of fetus between 24 to 32 weeks?

- 24th week – The fetus continues to grow and its vital organs are sufficiently mature. It is unlikely to maintain an independent life. The arms and legs have normal amount of muscle. The length of the fetus is 33 cms and it weighs 570 gm.

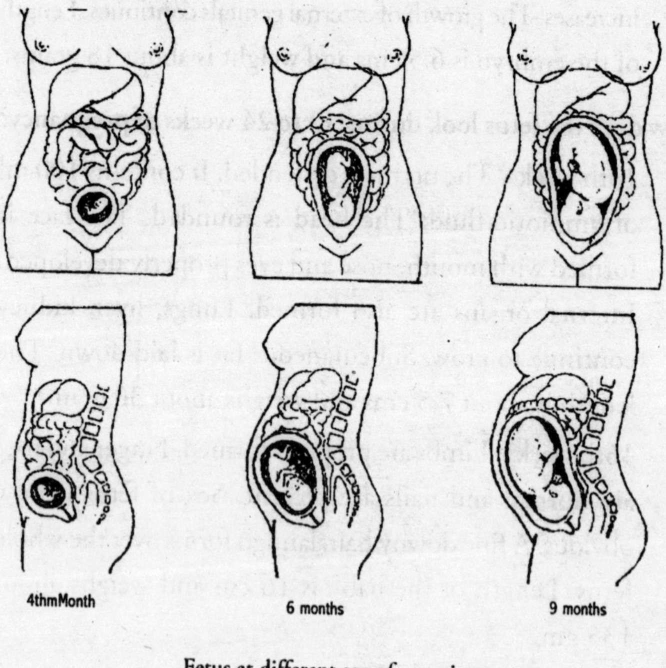

Fetus at different age of gestation

- 28th week – The fetus is now viable and can survive separately. Chances of survival are 75%. Before the 28th week termination of pregnancy is abortion. The fetus is now covered with vernix, which is a greasy, adhesive cheese like material. The length is 37 cms and weight is 900 grams.
- 32nd week – The child is perfectly formed. The amount of subcutaneous fat is increasing. The weight is 1.6 kg. The length is 40.5 cms.

What happens between the 36th - 40th weeks of pregnancy?

- 36th week – The baby is fully mature and chances of survival are 95 percent. Lungs may not be fully developed.
- 40th week – The baby is fully developed to be delivered. Fine hair has disappeared. The body is covered entirely with vernix. The nails are soft and will not damage the skin.

What is fetal lie?

It is the long axis of the fetus to the long axis of mother. It can be detected by finding two poles of fetus. The fetal head is usually harder and round than the large diffuse soft bottom of fetus. A line drawn between these two poles is known as axis.

LABOUR AND DELIVERY

Is it best to have a baby delivered in a hospital?

It is true that normal childbirth is a natural event and not a sickness. Delivery can take place at home also but a hospital delivery has certain advantages.

- A hospital can provide emergency services such as blood transfusion and surgery.
- No responsibility of preparing equipment, bed etc. for the delivery.
- The new mother can be trained by nurse.

How do you know that the labour has started?

The woman may suddenly feel energetic. There may be an intermittent low backache, deep in the pelvis. She starts contractions at 15-20 minutes intervals and these are strong.

There will be 'show' and rupture of membranes. Mucus comes out as a blood streaked discharge. Rupture of membranes may result in a sudden rush of liquid.

Is there any thing like false labour?

Over eager women can translate mild contractions into labour pain. It generally happens in the first delivery.

What happens in labour?

After 266-280 days the fetus has to be pushed out through a narrow bony outlet. Labour is the gradual process that enables the journey to be made.

What is the first stage of labour?

This is the longest and the most difficult during which the cervix has to be stretched. It lasts from the onset to dilatation of the cervix. This stage lasts for 10-12 hours in the first delivery and in later pregnancy time is reduced. Contractions come every 10-15 minutes and last 20-30 seconds. As the labour progresses contractions come at a shorter interval.

What happens in the second stage of labour?

This is the expulsive stage from full dilatation of cervix to the delivery of the baby. In the first delivery it lasts for an hour or so. Subsequently it becomes much shorter i.e. a few minutes, when the baby's head reaches the floor of the pelvis and starts to distend vaginal opening you will feel to bear down and push. Contractions are often still hard. As the head emerges

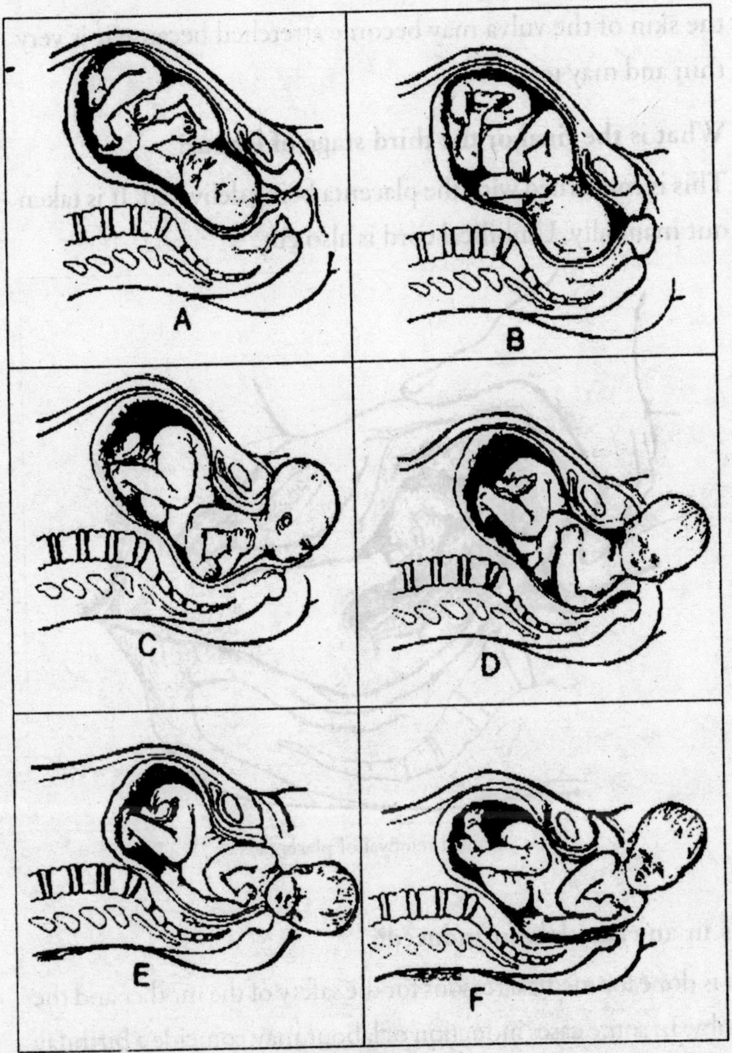

Process of delivery

the skin of the vulva may become stretched because it is very thin and may tear.

What is the final or the third stage of labour?

This is concerned with the placenta being delivered. It is taken out manually. Umbilical cord is also cut.

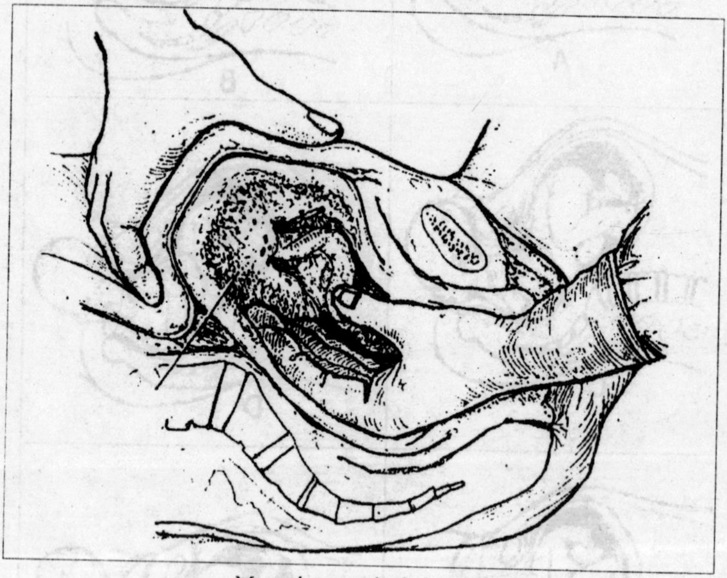

Manual removal of placenta

Is in any case labour induced?

It is done for medical reasons for the safety of the mother and the baby. In some cases induction of labour may coincide a birthday or a particular star sign. Medical reasons include prolonged labour, high blood pressure due to toxemia and fetal distress.

Syntocin drip helps.

What is episiotomy?

It is a procedure of deliberate cutting of skin behind the vaginal opening to help in the delivery of baby's head because the skin is too rigid to allow the head to come down. In fetal distress also it helps. A small cut is made and repairing a deliberate cut is simpler than stitching a ragged tear. Disadvantage of it is discomfort due to scar formation.

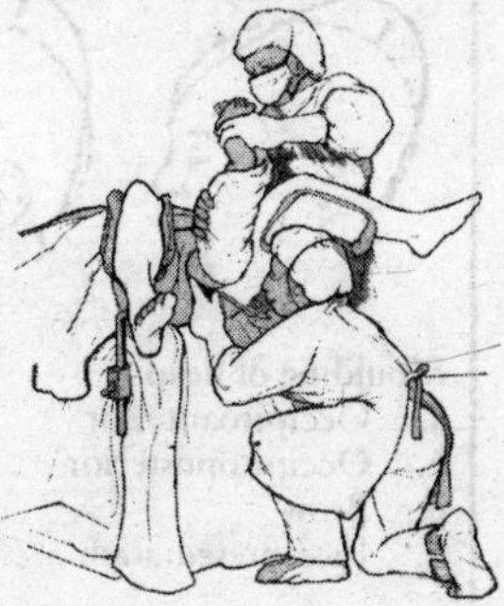

What do you understand by forceps delivery?

Forceps are essentially tongs, an instrument capable of helping in delivery without injury to the child or to the mother. Two blades of forceps fit accurately over the baby's head and then the head is taken out.

What do you understand by fetal distress?

Fetal distress is manifested by irregular or slow heart because the placenta provides less oxygen to the child. Prolapse of cord, premature separation of placenta may simply have exhausted the unborn baby.

Secondly there may be a delay in the second stage of labour. In breech presentation also forceps may be applied. Forceps delivery is never done in a hurry.

What is moulding of head?

It occurs in normal delivery to allow some degree of adjustment to pressure.

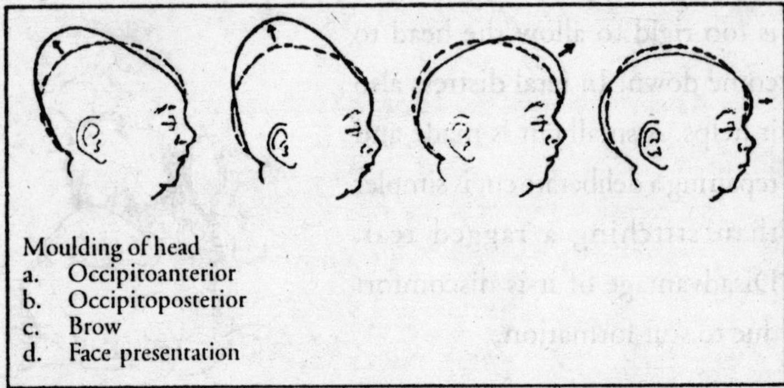

Moulding of head
a. Occipitoanterior
b. Occipitoposterior
c. Brow
d. Face presentation

Can placenta previa be serious?

It is the organ which supplies mother's blood to fetus. It is attached firmly to the lining of womb. By the end of pregnancy it is 8 inches wide and 1 inch thick. It acts as organ of respiration and excretion of fetus. It produces

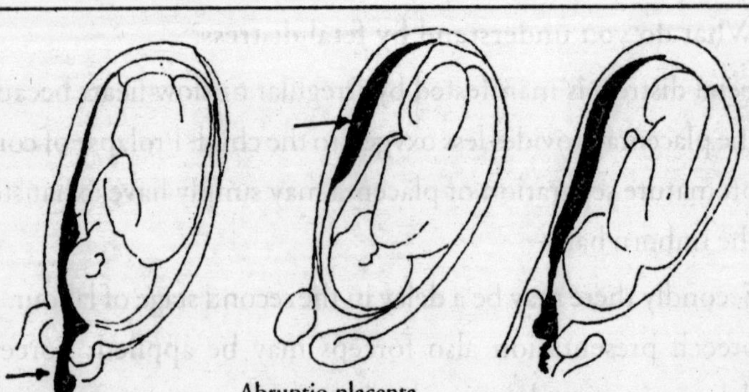

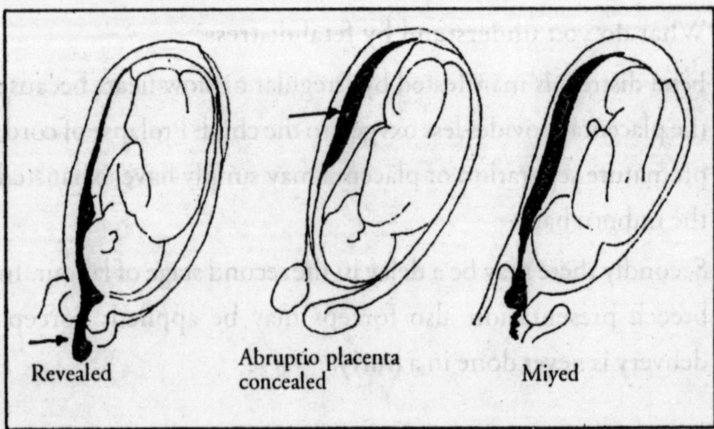

Revealed
Abruptio placenta concealed
Miyed

three hormones estrogen, progesterone and chronic gonadotropin. When attachment of placenta is lower down it may result in painless bleeding due to pressure of fetus parts.

What is lochia?

It is a veginal discharge that follows child birth and consist of blood and necrotic decidual, Lochia alba is white in colour from 9th to 15th day and is creamy in colour. Lochia rubra is

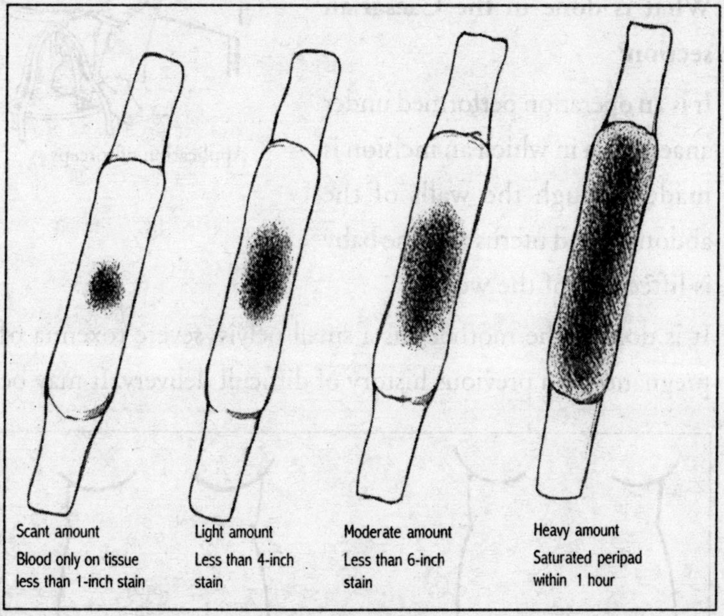

Peripad method

red in colour between 4th to 8th day. It contains shreds of decidual fragments.

What about complications from a forceps delivery?

- Occasionally there may be small tears in the vagina.
- There may be forceps marks over the head of the baby.
- Excessive tracking with difficult delivery may cause some bruising over the scalp and rarely permanent neurological effects.

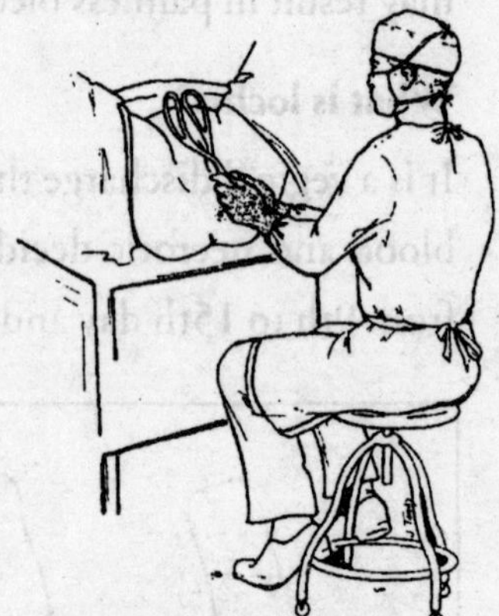

Application of forceps

What is done in the Caesarian section?

It is an operation performed under anaesthesia in which an incision is made through the walls of the abdomen and uterus and the baby is lifted out of the womb.

It is done if the mother has a small pelvis, severe toxemia of pregnancy or a previous history of difficult delivery. It may be

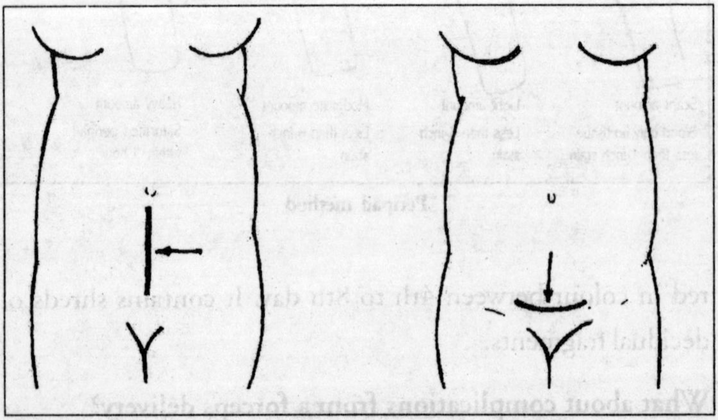

recommended if the placenta lies in front of the presenting part. From the baby's point of view this operation is considered safe. The incision may be vertical or horizontal.

What about post operative recovery?

After surgery there is a certain amount of discomfort for the first two or three days. Some pain may be felt under the shoulder blades. The pain or discomfort is usually relieved by sedatives and pain relievers.

Usually once a caesarian always a caesarian.

What is involution of uterus?

It is the process by which uterus regains its nonpregnant stage after delivery. Immediately after delivery uterus is 8 x 4½ inches. Thickness of body is ½ inches while at the end of puerperium it remains only 3 x 2 x 1 inches. The involution is produced by the process of autolysis.

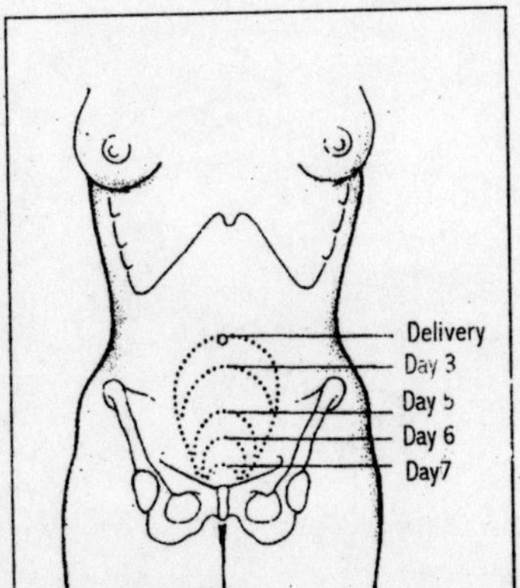

Involution of uterus

BREAST FEEDING

Many of the modern mothers don't want to breast feed their children as they fear that they will lose the consistency and contour of their charm

What is the economics of breast feeding?

Milk secreted by Indian mothers has been noted to be about 600 ml the cost of which will be about eight rupees per day. In six months you will spend 1500/- to about 2500/- if child is given bottle feed. If all the women of Asia were to cease breast feeding an extra herd of 114,000,000 cattles will be needed to make good this loss.

What are the advantages of breast feeding?

- It provides the baby with milk of a suitable composition and correct temperature.
- It provides a warm happy relationship between the mother and the child.

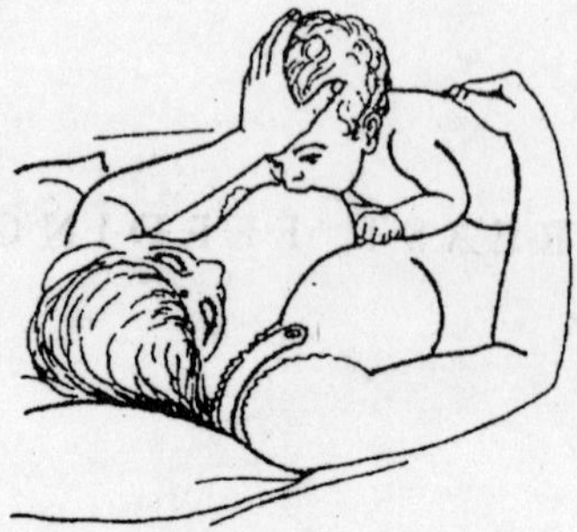

- There is no risk of the contamination of milk during the process of feeding.
- It helps in involution i.e. coming back of the pregnant uterus to the normal position.
- No sterilization is required. Breast feeding can be done, at any place and time.
- It does not result in any loose motions or any other infection.

What is colostrum?

The yellowish secretion from the breasts during the first 2-3 days after delivery is known as colostrum. It has a high protein and vitamin A content and confers an immunity against infections during the first few months. It also helps in the development and production of enzyme required for digestion.

What is the composition of various types of milk?

Composition of milk per 100 gm

Nutrient	Human milk	Cow's milk	Buffalo's milk	Goat's milk
Protein gm	1.1	3.2	4.3	3.3
Fat gm	3.4	4.1	8.8	4.5
Calcium (mg)	28	120	210	170
Iron (mg)	0.2	0.2	0.3	
Vitamin C (mg)	03	02	01	01
Vitamin A (mg)	42	52	48	54
Calories	65	67	117	72

Does mother's milk give protection against allergy?

When the new born infant is fed on marketed food an allergic reaction can be set up. People with an allergic history in the family such as asthma or eczema or food disagreement are advised to give their babies only breast milk.

What are the long term benefits of breast feeding?

The children will be less likely to develop heart disease and complaints of digestive tract. Breast fed babies will hardly become obese. They are unlikely to suffer from tooth decay. Their sucking mechanism is healthier.

How to prepare nipples for breast feeding?

When the baby first sucks, it moves the nipples in a completely new way. They may be pulled out and stretched forcibly and repeatedly and they are sometimes chewed resulting in soreness, cracks and even oozing blood. To avoid this during the last days of pregnancy the woman should pull out her nipples with her fingers, stretching them as much as possible without hurting them. A dozen pullings at each nipple everyday should help to accustom the nipples to the sucking action.

What should be the position of the mother and child during breast feeding?

The mother should hold the baby close enough to her body for its chin to touch her breast all the time. If the baby is not close enough to the breast it may have to suck too hard on the nipples in order to keep it in his mouth. This excess suction can damage the sensitive nipple skin. A baby must be held close enough to the breast to keep the nipple and the areola in place inside its mouth without much effort.

Why is there an early breast engorgement?

When milk first comes in breasts, one may feel full and uncomfortable. Some women may have painful stony hard engorged breasts. A brief spike of fever may occur at this time. It is known as milk fever.

These symptoms are due to increased amount of blood and tissue fluid in the breast. Simple answer to this problem is to express the milk manually, because if the breast is engorged the nipple may be stretched flat and not easily protactile. The baby can only chew at the tip of the nipple and cannot suck properly.

What to do in case of sore nipples?

- Frequent short feedings promote speedy healing.
- Let the baby suck on the affected breast first. Because initial sucking is the strongest and most painful.
- If both sides are equally painful then very careful hand milking may elicit the ejection reflex and then the baby can be put to breasts when the milk starts flowing.
- Mother can apply a thin coat of edible oil. Never apply tincture of benzoin or spirit.

What to do when breasts starts leaking?

Lack of tone of sphincter muscle around the milk ducts causes a steady leakage. Using pieces of cloth or absorbent paper in the brassiere or clothes are worn over the breasts is the obvious solution. These pieces must be clean, dried and must be changed frequently.

Sometimes when the baby is feeding at one breast, milk flows from the other. For this the mother can press one finger over the unsuckled nipple.

Why a baby cries too much?

Cry of an infant is a signal to world, a plea for contact. Some infants remain angry and discontented, may be that he is getting too little a milk. A long sound sleep after breast feed shows that the feed was sufficient in quantity.

Why do some children vomit after the feed?

Many babies regurgitate some milk when they bring 'wind' or if they have taken a large feed. Vomited part is very minimal and the feed is mixed with saliva and other intestinal fluids. If the baby is feeding well and gaining weight then need not to worry.

What is the relation of mothers milk to her diet?

- Lactation seems to be physiologically well protected so that it does not decline as fast as woman's diet decreases.
- Milk production is maintained at the expense of woman's reserve.
- Milk from well nourished women and from women with specific nutritional deficiencies does not differ much nutritionally.
- Even under seriously adverse nutritional conditions human milk is uniquely valuable to the baby.
- The mother requires about 620 extra calories to produce 800 ml of milk. She may secret 10 gm per day high quality protein. Additional 20 gram protein to a normal diet is recommended to compensate it.

When is the manual expression of milk indicated?

Expressing milk is useful in a number of situations

- For the relief of the engorgement of the breast.
- To continue feeding a sick or low birth baby.
- To help maintain a milk supply when nursing is interrupted due to some reason.
- To store the feed when the mother wants to go away.

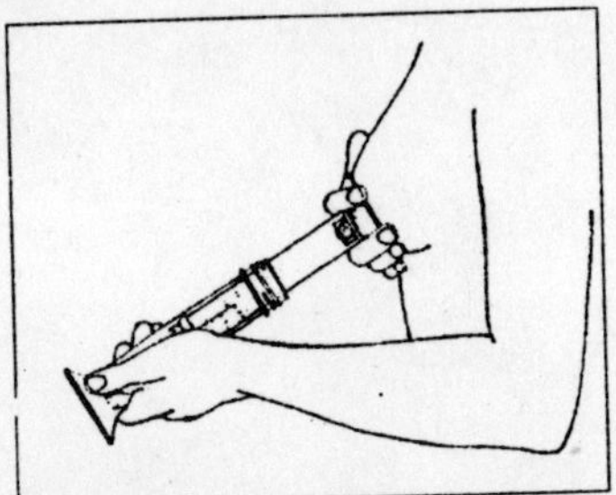

Manual expression of breast milk

Which drugs are contraindicated while nursing?

Following drugs may not be taken

- Radio iodine
- Anticancer drugs
- Heroin
- Lithium
- Chloramphenicol

Which drugs should be avoided while nursing?

- Diazepam
- Barbiturate
- Tetracyclines
- Nalidixic acid
- Metronidazole
- Steroids

Prenatal exercise

1. **Palvic floor exercises** – Lying down on back, legs apart and chest relaxed.

   Draw up the pelvic floor. Squeeze the vagina and place one hand over the pubic bones and think about tightening the birth canal as high as possible. Hold for 2-3 seconds and relax. Do only 2-3 times.

2. **Abdominal tightening** – Lying on back.,knees bent, place

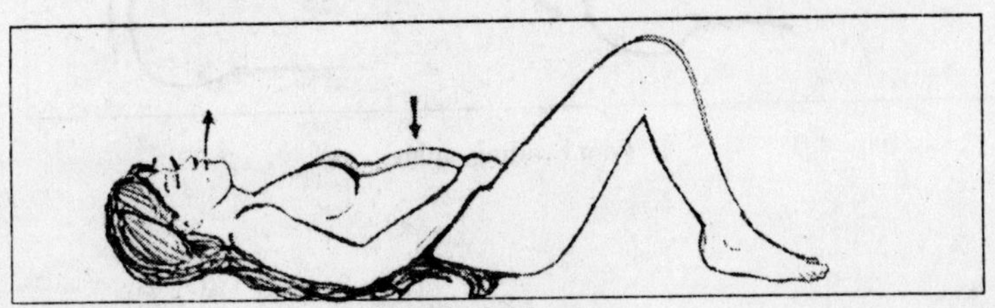

Abdominal tightening

your hands on lower abdomen.

Take a deep complete breath through nose. Keep the ribs still and let the abdominal wall expand upward. Then blow the air through mouth slowly and forcibly pulling in your abdominal muscles. Action is like blowing a trumpet.

3. **Foot bending and foot stretching** – It helps in return of blood from lower legs and will minimise and swelling of ankles. Cramps may be minimised.

Sitting or lying bend the ankle as for as you can. Pull

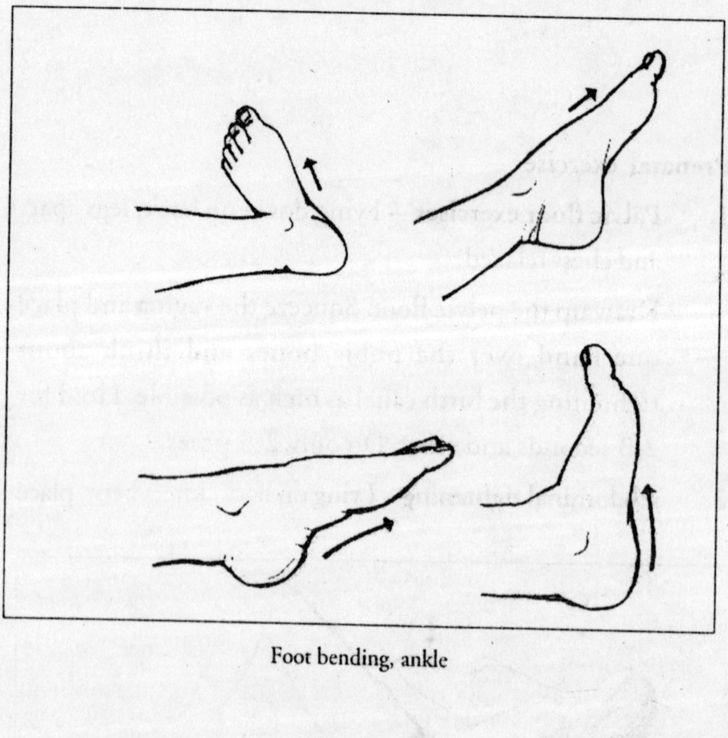

Foot bending, ankle

your toes upwards stretching the calf muscles. Then point the foot downward making an arch. Do this several times.

4. **Pelvic tilting** – Lie on your back with knees bent. Roll the pelvis back by flattening the lower back down on

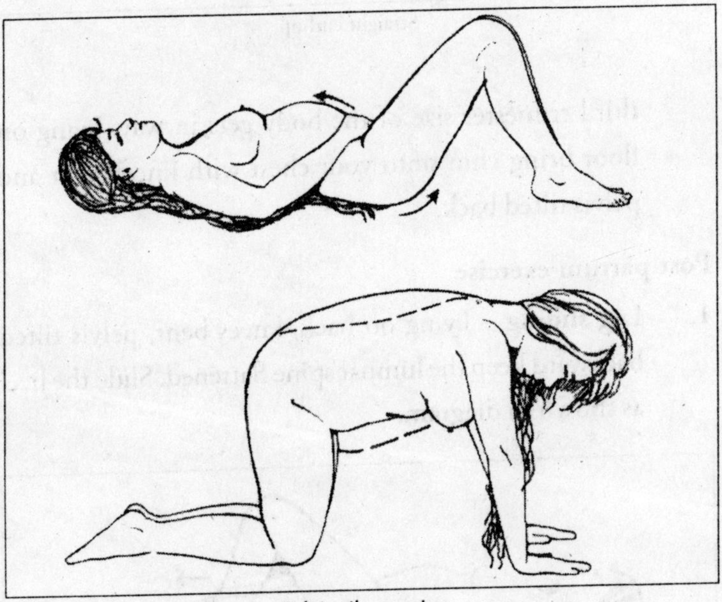

Pelvic tilt exercise

the floor. To strengthen action place a hand just above the pubic bone so that you can feel the muscles working.

5. **Straight curl up** – This exercise is for starters. During

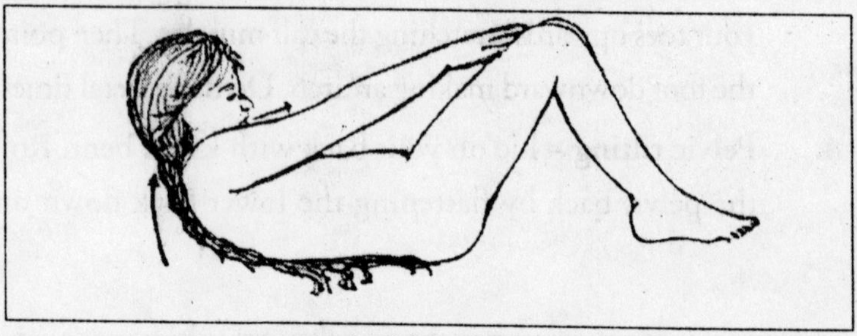

Straight curl up

third trimester size of the body gets in way. Lying on floor bring chin onto your chest with knees bent and pelvis tilted back.

Post partum exercise

1. **Leg sliding** – Lying on back, knees bent, pelvis tilted backward keep the lumbar spine flattened. Slide the heel as shown in diagram.

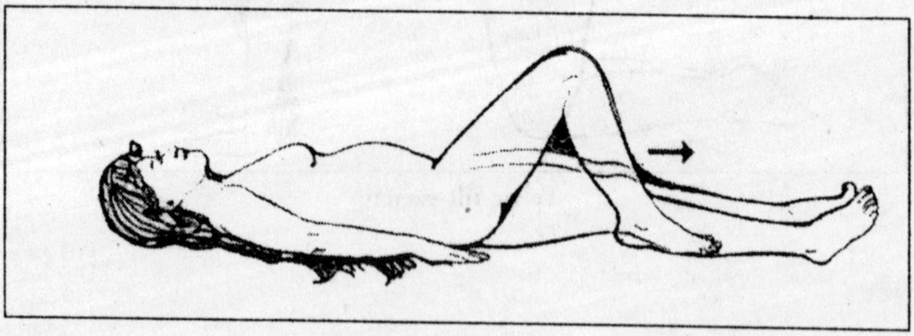

Leg sliding

2. **Diagonal curl up** – Lying on back with knees bent bring your chin onto your chest. As you breath out fold forward

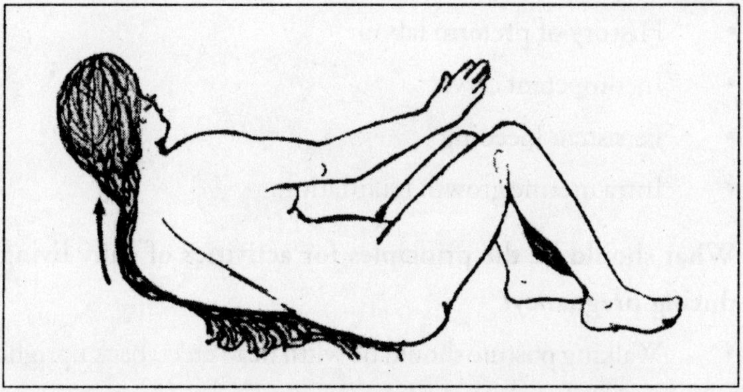

Diagonal curl up

reaching with your out stretched arm to the left knee. Slowly return back to your original position.

What are warning signs and symptoms during or after exercise?

If lady develops following signs exercise has to be discontinued immediately

- Pain
- Bleeding
- Shortness of breath
- Palpitation.
- Faintness
- Increase of pulse
- Back/Pubic pain

When is exercise not to be done?

In following conditions exercise should not be done.

- Pregnancy induced hypertension
- Preterm rupture of membranes

- History of preterm labour
- Incompetent cervix
- Persistent bleeding
- Intra uterine growth retardation.

What should be the principles for activities of daily living during pregnancy?

- Walking posture should be wiith head erect, back upright and abdomen tucked
- Use a foot stool when sitting
- When climbing stairs, the entire foot should be placed on stair. Leg muscles should be used to lift self up with each step without leaning forward.
- Stooping and lifting should be avoided. When it is necessary it is best to squat down and reach and lift with feet wide apart and back straight.
- When carrying bulky package, load should be balanced putting infront if possible.

What are the breathing techniques for birth?

During second state of labour

- Don't strain. Let go and flow with contraction.

* Relax the pelvic floor. Don't tense the muscles when you feel rectal pressure.

* Increase the pressure on abdomen and not on your face.

- Avoid prolonged pushes which affect your breathing.

INFERTILITY

What do you understand by infertility?

The desire for reproduction is a basic human attribute and infertility causes distress in many Indian couples. Fertility is maximum in the mid twenties and in women it declines after the age of 30. Intercourse twice a week seems minimum for a reasonable chance of success and a high rate of pregnancy has been reported after coital frequencies of 4 or more times weekly. In absence of contraceptives about 60% of women will become pregnant in first 6 months of marriage, 80% within first year.

What should be the purpose of infertility investigations?

The purpose of infertility investigations are –

- to offer an explanation for the infertility
- to decide on mode of treatment

to give a prognosis whether they can have a child or not?

10% couples are infertile even without any cause.

What investigations should be done in case of a male?

Unless the husband is willing to co-operate fully, it is futile to investigate only female.

On taking the history questions should be asked about childhood disease of mumps or orchitis, exposure of radioactive substances, consumption of tobacco/alcohol and sexual habits including knowledge of anatomy of coitus, impotence and premature ejaculation.

Congenital abnormalities such as hypospadias or cryptorchism should be noted. Failure of descent of testes leads to azoospermia.

What about examining of sperm in case of infertility?

The patient should abstain from sex for several days before collection of semen. The specimen is obtained by masturbation and is collected in a sterile glass jar. Rubber or plastic container should not be used. Laboratory examination is to be done within first 2 hours. A normal specimen measures more than 2 ml and contains 20,00000 sperms per ml. More than 60% sperms should be motile and less than 25% of abnormal forms. Poor mobility or numerous abnormal sperm forms are of more serious significance than a low count. If count is very less, estimation of FSH, LH, testosterone and thyroid function test should be done. Sometimes testicular biopsy may be of help.

What clear advise is to be given to males?

Advise should be given to the husband on conclusion of all necessary investigations. Where there is reasonable hope of fertility encouragement should be given. If he is hopelessly infertile he should be told clearly.

What are the normal values of semen analysis?

Volume	2-5 ml
Liquefaction	complete in 20-30 minutes
Count	>20 million per ml
Motility	>60% motile after one hour
	>50% mobile after 2 hours
WBCs	None
Bacteria	None to a few

Can dysparunia and vaginismus be cause of infertility?

Pain during sex and difficulty in penetration will not allow a perfect coitus. It is more of a psychological problem and putting cervical dilators may be helpful.

What can be the role of cervix in infertility?

To achieve fertilization the sperm has to pass through the cervix. Cervical mucus acts as a barrier to sperm except around the time of ovulation when mucus is translucent and thin.

Post coital test is the only method which examines both partners simultaneously. There may be cervical mucus hostility. It may occur when mucus may be deficient, unduely thick or lethal to sperm. Sperm penetration of cervical mucus may be improved by giving oestrogen for a week before ovulation.

What are the uterine causes resulting in infertility?

Various forms of duplicacy and retroverted uterus can cause it. Fibroids may also cause gross distortion of uterine cavity but on occasions multiple fibroids are seen in pregnancy.

Hystero salpingography with a radio opaque dye is the best way of study of uterus.

How does endometrial biopsy help?

The most important disease diagnosed by endometrial biopsy is T.B. It is always due to tuberculous salpingitis and prognosis of fertility is poor.

Is study of fallopian tubes necessary in case of infertility?

Fallopian tubes are the channels through which ovum is transferred to uterus. Ampulla or fimbria pick up the ovum. It is then transported by cilia to the site of fertilization. The zygote is nourished and matured and finally transported to uterine cavity. Many cases of sterility are caused by blockage of Fallopian tubes by inflammation. Laparoscopy is now the initial investigation of tubal function.

How ovaries play part in infertility?

Ovaries show evidence of inadequate function in 10 to 15 percent infertile females, who either fail to ovulate at all or have an inadequate leuteal phase. Ultrasound provides interesting, direct and atraumatic method of observing the physical changes in the ovary with ovulation.

Serial measurement of ovary throughout the cycle shows increasing follicular diameters to about 20 m.m. before ovulation followed by a sharp decrease thereafter.

Polycystic ovary syndrome may result in infertility.

What are the non medical factors of inhibiting fertility?

Sometimes couples may engage in sexual habits and preferences that are inadvertently detrimental to conception. The use of lubricants such as petroleum jelly and water soluble lubricant jelly during coitus may inhibit sperm motality or actually serve as a spermicide.

The use of post coital douches or the act of woman rising immediately after intercourse may remove semen pool from vagina. Woman should be advised to remain supine for 30 minutes after intercourse to allow semen pool to reach the cervix.

Premature ejaculation may inhibit fertility because semen is not correctly placed in vagina to reach the cervix. This condition can be reversed with specific exercises and alternative position for coitus.

Financial stress, frustration, fatigue may influence fertility. Some couples may not be doing sex during ovulation period when female is most fertile or they are unable to complete intercourse because of female anatomical malformations that prevent full penetration due to rigid perineal body or vaginismus.

What is donor artificial insemination?

This is the successful form of treatment of male subfertility. Fresh semen has a 70% success rate of 12 months. Sperm donors are usually unknown to female recipient and are screened

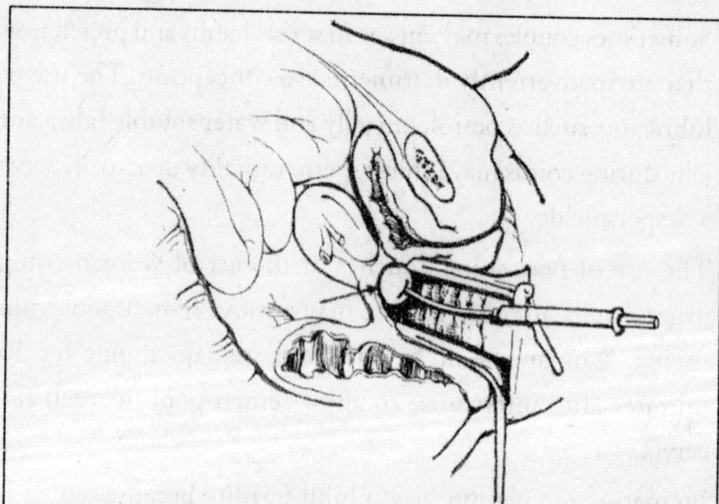

Artificial insemination

for genetic diseases and for AIDS. Recipient must be in her time of ovulation. Donors may be carefully matched to some of husbands physical characteristics including hair, eye colour, body built and IQ.

Can there be an artificial insemination by husband?

The treatment success is only 6-20%. It is used mainly for couples who find donor insemination ethically unacceptable.

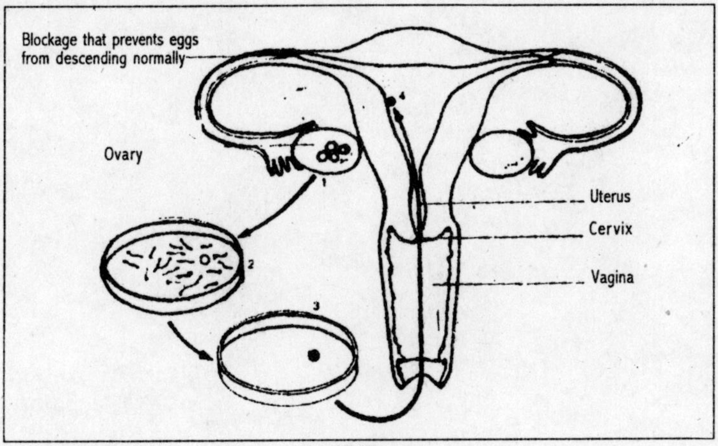

IVF
Invitro fertilisation

Highest success rate occur if infertility is caused by impotence, hypospadias, retrograde ejaculation or cervical mucus hostility. Concentrating the sperms of men with poor counts don't improve pregnancy chances.

Joy of Sex

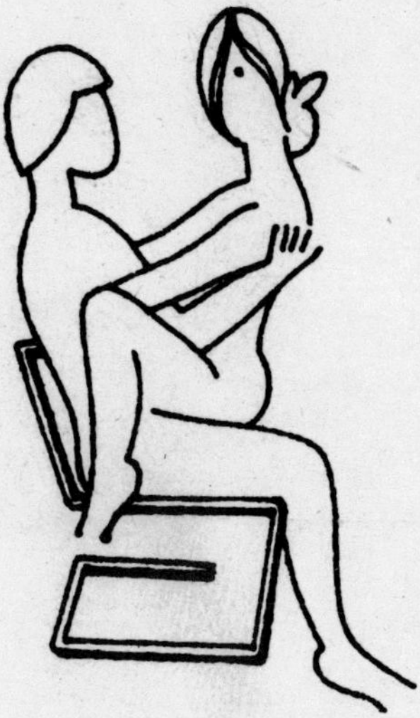

Joy of Sex

L C Gupta, M.D., D.Sc
Kusum Gupta, (Eng. Lit.) Ph.D

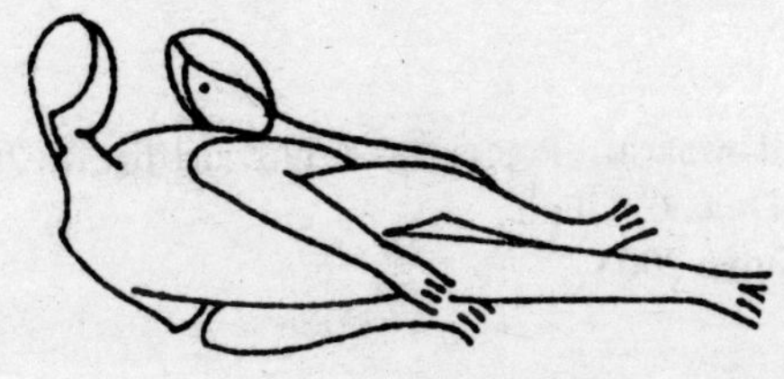

Srishti
PUBLISHERS & DISTRIBUTORS

Srishti Publishers & Distributors
64-A, Adhchini
Sri Aurobindo Marg
New Delhi 110 017
srishtipublishers@yahoo.com

First published by Srishti Publishers & Distributors in 2003

ISBN 81-88575-16-x

Typeset in AGaramond 11pt. by Skumar at Srishti

PREFACE

Sex drive is a natural aspect of life which needs to be both understood and controlled. It should be considered as a meaningful and respectable part of married life. The goal o sexuality is to love, mate, reproduce and care for the young ones.

Sexual adjustment is a part of the individual's total development into maturity. Sexual maturity brings out what is best, most generous and most constructive in life.

Sex education leads to decreased sexual experimentation. Provision of information about various aspects of sexuality is necessary to help young people make empowered decisions so that they can protect themselves from abuse, infection and unwanted conception.

When, where, how and how much to tell and by whom are a matter of debate. But there is a need to give correct information with a proper sense of values. The eager curiosity if guided properly will give them a high standard of moral behaviour saving them from emotional pit falls.

Giving knowledge of sex is like unfolding of spring, predictive and repetitive yet nonetheless enchanting.

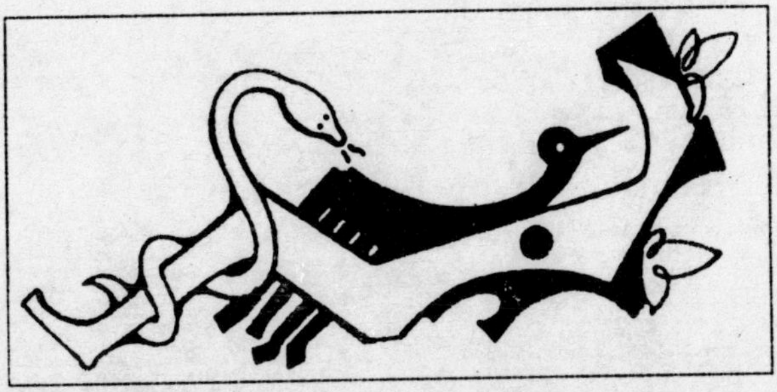

CONTENTS

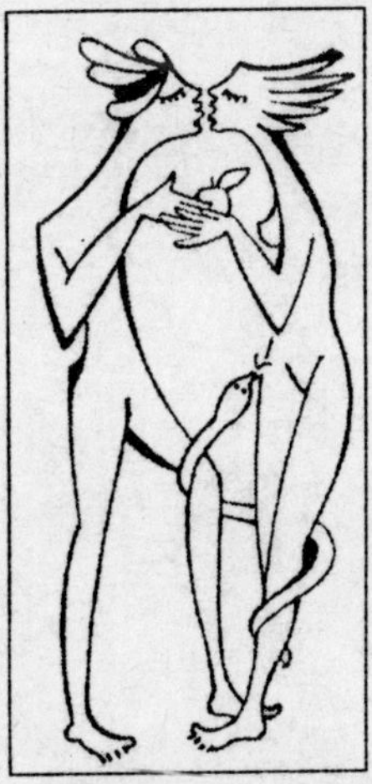

SEX & MARRIAGE

What is marriage?

Sex and the event of child bearing are considered so essential for family life that couples staying together without marriage, the single parent and childless families are not accepted as complete or normal families.

What is the role of marriage in society?

Marriage is a contract between a man and a woman to live together preferably till life. Reproduction may be the main aim but sex plays a prominent role in marriage and a satisfying relationship is a must for a happy union. However a lasting relationship cannot be based merely on sexual attraction.

Are the joys of sex and reproduction two different things?

The spread of birth control knowledge has made separation of sex from reproduction. It has realised more dynamic sex expression in marriage. New cultural and economic changes have forced a re-evaluation and reappraisal of former sex ethics and standards.

Is sex simply an instinct?

Instinct is an innate tendency to behave in a specific manner as a result of certain stimuli. From childhood we are subjected to restrictions, suppression and taboos which affect our normal sex instincts and condition us against a natural sex expression. After marriage it requires a conscious and intelligent effort for its realization. In man the actual technique to bring satisfaction in sex is a learned process. This requires first of all an understanding of the mechanism involved in sex and sexual love.

Is dynamic sex a natural gift?

Harmonious and dynamic sex does not develop automatically but it needs an understanding of nature and the mechanism of sex union. This you pick up after some observation and experience only.

It is also true that successful marriage can hardly be attained without sexual attraction.

What factors have led to the present day change in women's attitude towards sex?

Growing independence of women have enabled them to exercise greater freedom and initiative in the choice of a partner and in the expression of their sexual needs.

Is knowledge of anatomy and physiology of sex organs necessary?

It makes you wiser if you have the knowledge of the mechanism involved in the sex of genital organs, changes occurring in sexual stimulation and excitation. It is also desirable that couples should know the physiology of coitus too.

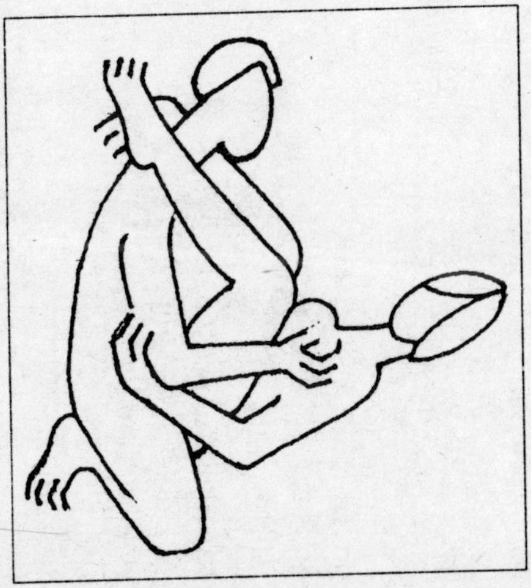

SEX AS A HEALTH PROMOTER

Phenylethylamine, is a brain chemical which closely resembles amphetamine. It energises your body keeping you on a high. Touch between lovers boosts a hormone called oxytocin secreted by the pituitary gland. When oxytocin is generated it increases our desire to be touched boosting the further release of hormone oxytocin making us want to hug, kiss and cuddle. It works with the female hormone estrogen so its effect is greater in women.

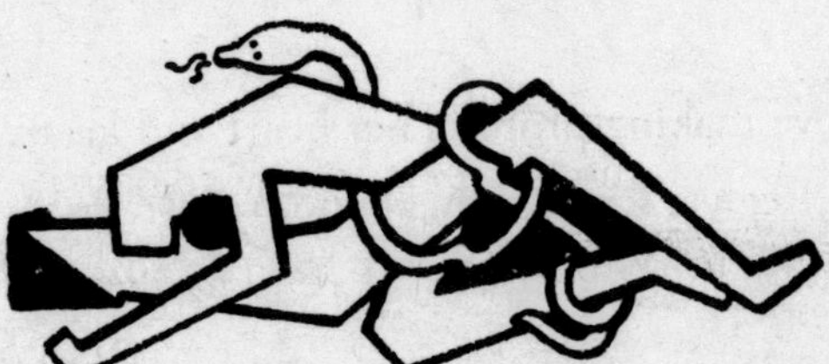

Can sex relieve pain?

When some women climax a natural pain blocker is released in the spinal cord. Vaginal stimulation blocks the release of neurotransmitter 'P' which is responsible of conveying our sensation of pain to the brain. Sex is a perfect way to relieve headache due to endorphins released during coitus.

Can sex be helpful in releasing stress?

Sex and stress trigger similar physiological reactions. Heart rate and blood pressure rises, respiration quickens, pupils dilate and the pain threshold rises.

Having sex can suffuse both partners with a profound feeling of well being and relaxation reducing the stress level.

What other benefits are there of the sexual activity?

One successful act burns about 150-300 calories in young age and about 100 calories after the age of 60. If you can have sex three times a week in a year you spend more than 15, to 20,000 calories which is equivalent of jogging 150-200 miles.

It keeps your cholesterol level lower and rises the level of HDL a good cholesterol. The testosterone released during sex fortifies bones and muscles.

A woman's regular love making protects her heart and keeps vaginal tissues supple. Regular sex, regulates periods and reduces premenstrual tension.

What is the relationship between sexual activity and health of the prostate?

In the case of male most prostate problems start in old age when the fluids of glands are not emptied out efficiently. Sex is a simple remedy for it. During orgasm the muscles around the prostate contract on several occasions squeezing the excess fluid. Regular sex is therefore important for continued prostate health.

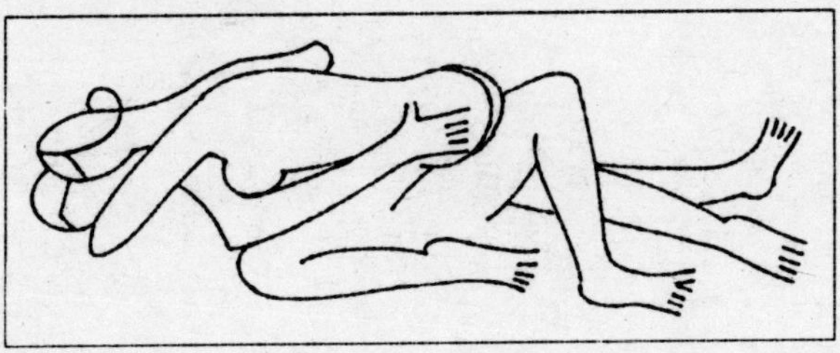

SEX GUIDE FOR EVERY DECADE

Sex matures with age. You should know that your sex desire and performance works differently with every decade.

What about sexual activity during teenage?

You may not be enjoying sex because you don't know the philosophy and chemistry of it. What you know is the physical act and attraction only.

What about the third decade?

Your sexual appetite is growing upward with age, you will like to attain orgasm. You become more assertive and more demanding in bed.

Don't jump into the bed as soon as husband arrives. Let the preliminaries i.e. holding hand, cuddling, kissing, necking, petting be an appetiser.

If you are intimate in conversation you will find more intimacy in bed.

What happens in the 4th decade?

Oestrogen begins to fluctuate but not the sexual desire because testosterone controls the sex drive in both sexes.

Your menstrual periods may become irregular. You may start hot flushes and the vagina may dry. Look at your partner from a new angle and exchange fantasies.

What about sex in the fifties?

Period comes to a hault. Vaginal lining thins out and the vagina itself shrinks to cause painful sex. Depression may result due to lack of sex.. But some females find it more satisfying because children don't disturb and there is no fear of pregnancy.

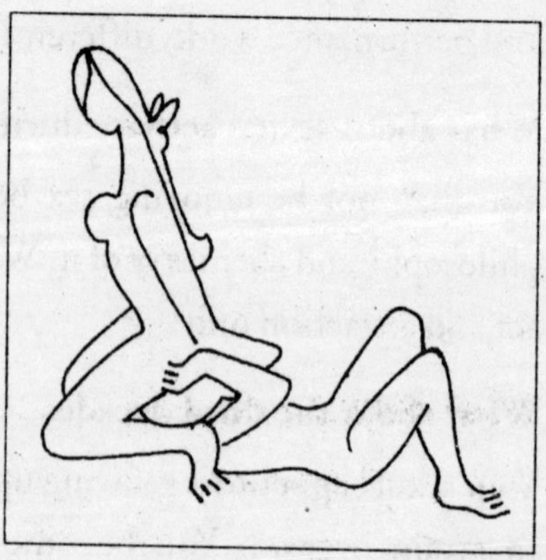

THE BRIDAL NIGHT

What is marital relationship?

Having been strenuously trained all their lives to avoid all persons of opposite sex except members of their family, it is impossible for a young married couple to be at ease with each other at the start of marriage. Months pass before a young husband is able to speak to his wife without shame and embarrassment, under such circumstances she should work closely with her mother in-law and sister in law to become a new daughter in their house.

What about virginity?

The Bride is expected to be a virgin and the husband is delighted when he finds his wife's hymen to be unperforated. However there may be lack of bleeding after the first intercourse. Many a virgin may not have hymen. Certain social activities like sports, cycling may tear the hymen. Despite the value placed on early sexual continence it is not virginity as such that is valued, instead chastity before marriage reveals a girl to be morally sound and reliable hence as a wife she is less likely to be an adultress and a worry to her husband.

What is the importance of the first kiss?

The First kiss is the most memorable experience of one's life. It is so powerful that these romantic movements are recalled very precisely. Couples can recall details of kiss even site, environment and even the dress they wore at that moment. It is more romantic than one's losing of virginity. In losing the virginity the factor of anxiety is there of becoming pregnant.

What is the secret of good kissing?

The secret of good kissing is in its variety. So one should try and inject as many emotions as one can. Be considerate about the desire of the partner.

There is nothing worse than kissing a partner with a bad breath. One can use a mouth freshner.

Timing is one of the important factors while kissing. It may be after petting and a friendly pack. Start out by slow kissing after getting the response, go ahead with lips.

How do other family members behave with a new daughter-in-law?

In a marriage a husband gets a wife but at least for a few months she becomes a centre of attraction for other young members of the family too. For some she is a 'dear bhabhi' to have fun with.

Elders are also very considerate and provide a separate room to the new couple well decorated and perfumed with flowers so that the couple can learn to grow fond of each other and to develop an easy intimacy. Here the couple has privacy to gratify their sexual and other personal relations.

Is coitus necessary on bridal night?

Not necessarily. For the first few days husband and wife should talk and have fun and try to know each other to develop emotionally for having a successful act.

Is sexual act on the first night painful?

Any pain if experienced is due to the actual stretching or breaking of the hymen. In most cases it is thin and elastic and will give way, but in rare cases if it is firm and tense then the entry will give pain. Relaxation of wife helps. Rigidity of muscles makes it more difficult.

Even if the first coitus is painful should the husband continue the act?

No, if the entry is very painful or if there is much apprehension and fear on the part of wife, complete penetration need not take place. Prolonged foreplay will relax the woman and sufficient lubrication will ease the discomfort. It will also decrease the anxiety of the woman.

What is the importance of the first sexual experience?

Successful first sex encounter relaxes the female and gives the confidence. Even if the first encounter is uncomfortable it is not advisable to put off the consumation. When her coitus is postponed for a longer time the greater will be the anxiety on the part of wife and husband and they will develop frustration. It is true that cruelty, clumsiness and discomfort on the first night may make future adjustment more difficult .

Generally women find it difficult to yield to the sexual union because of modesty or due to their training and upbringing or due to fear of possible discomfort. They may even physically resist sex.

Does a woman enjoy sex on the first night?

A fairly high percentage of women don't react fully to the sexual embrace until some time, after sex the relation has been established, some may develop disappointment.

Intimacies during the premarital courtship tend to develop a feeling of confidence and trust and it lessens her resistance to sex and derives usual type of sexual satisfaction.

What do you understand by defloration?

The hymen surrounds the vaginal entrance and the male organ has to pass through it to enter the vaginal canal. The length of an erect penis is more than 6 inches and a diameter of about 1.5 inches. The pressure of the male organ first causes the hymen to stretch and may permit entry while continued pressure results in the breaking of membrane known as defloration.

Does a lot of blood come out during defloration?

No, blood is scanty not requiring any first aid and such spotting may recur during the first few relationships.

Previously bleeding was taken as a sign of virginity and as a proof a blood stained bed sheet used to be displayed to the neighbours the next morning.

Should any partner disclose having sex with some one else on the bridal night?

Never confess having sex with other men because even if your love is true husband will start thinking about your past, your character and feel totally shattered and he may start thinking of a break up. His thoughts may become obsessive in nature and threaten to ruin the relationship.

What does a woman like on the first night?

Woman may like flattery. A woman loves when her man touches her face lightly. Trace her cheeks with the finger tips upto ears. You can run your fingers through her hair.

Instead of penetration a woman wants romance, cuddling, hand holding and kissing. Women complain that their husbands don't touch them except in bed. A man should play with her fingers and hair.

Most women derive almost as much pleasure from physical closeness and emotional intimacy as from orgasm. Simply reaching orgasm without enjoying all this is like reaching a hill top on a helicopter without enjoying all the beauty of the landscape along the way.

What do you understand by touch?

Hugging, kissing, stroking, cuddling and embracing are some of the common ways to touch people with whom we share special bonds.

Touching and being touched are a physical expression of love that help a person acquire emotional maturity. Touch reactivates the chemistry of your body.

How an absence of touch affects human beings?

Indians actually speaking hesitate a lot when it comes to the display of physical love and affection. Even father does not kiss the young daughter and once she becomes an adult avoids touching her.

Maladjusted, emotionally unstable, insecure and cranky persons are those who have never been cuddled and hugged as children.

Can women differentiate between one touch and another?

All touches are not the same and an experienced girl can differentiate those easily. She knows when a touch on the butt conveys friendliness and when it amounts to a sexually suggestive gesture.

What is petting?

It is a sort of love making but stopping short of a sexual

intercourse. It is mostly prevalent in adolescent girls. In light petting or necking couples kiss passionately, clothed bodies are in contact of each other. But a girl may not allow the boy's wandering hands to palpate her vulva.

In heavy petting passionate kissing, love bites, breast stimulation takes place. Private parts may be fondled, ectasy may be achieved but technically girls still remain virgin. Petting plays an important role in the development of social behaviour as it offers emotional interaction and body exploration. It tells you about the magic of touch.

What is the role of honey moon?

A newly wed couple goes for a honey moon trip to a hill station near by or to some foreign country to enjoy.

There they are alone and get all twenty four hours at their disposal. Sexual union is both a physical and an emotional experience. To render a sexual embrace a pleasant experience to understand and appreciate each others reactions and feelings and to harmonize sex in day light as well during night hours, honey moon is an ideal. During honeymoon a couple becomes frank and gets the sufficient time to know each other emotionally and physically. Sexual activity is a shared experience neither a duty nor a routine of marriage.

Do husband and wife understand each others' sexual needs?

Too often couples fail to understand each others' needs. A husband should realise that the sexual desire of the woman requires a more sensitive and delicate approach while a wife generally doesn't understand the urgent sexual release of her husband and fails to cooperate and take active part in sex.

Does premarital sex give a better understanding of sex during honeymoon?

It will depend upon the nature and extent of the sexual experiences. If the sexual encounters are casual with call girls and prostitutes, it may not be fruitful. Courting of years is required to understand the chemistry of sex. While going to a prostitute a man obtains relief for himself and he does not arouse or gratify the woman nor does he understand her needs.

How does coitus in animals and human beings differ?

A certain amount of wooing and play prior to sex union has been seen in animals. Among animals coitus is not possible unless the female is willing to receive the male. The male has to persue the female and win her before she will accept him sexually. It is only in apes and man that sexual relations may take place even when the female has no desire for act.

Are there any set rules for sex play?

No, not at all. No form of sex play is wrong in itself unless it gives rise to physical injury or to undesirable emotional or aesthetic reactions. One should develop its own skill and make love a mutual adventure. It is necessary for the husband to evoke the desire in his wife to embrace coitus. She loves to be cared. Erogenous zones of a woman are more extensive and diverse, than man.

Can your jewellery be sensuous?

A newly wed wear a lot of jewellery. Jewellery is sensual in design and form. Soft necklaces, drooping earings are noticed easily. Sexy jewellery is more for the young. It can be elegant, natural and feminine. It is the design which makes a woman feel confident and sensuous.

Jewellery is a language. It is a form of expression which translates feeling of seduction and love through movements, shapes, colours and textures. Jewellery worn closest to the face adds the sparkle to the eyes. While jewellery worn as armbands or on ankles has a seductive appeal, coloured stones add to the aphrodisiac power.

How do joint families affect your sex life?

In a nuclear family or on honeymoon you are free to have physical contact the way you like. In a joint family a newcomer is circled by other family members during day hours and only the night is available for the new couple.

But the joint families in contrast to the nuclear ones are seen as providing support and comfort to the new member under stress. Inbuilt systems of joint family act as buffers against problems and cushion the affect of anxiety provoking events. Intelligent bhabhi acts as an advisor on sex matters to a new bride.

What is the sexual attitude of man towards the woman during a honeymoon?

Because women are trained to be obedient to men they are not expected to be able to refuse the sexual advances of a man. Man on the other hand feels it is the wife's duty to accept them whenever they ask, no matter how often, unless there is some serious physical reason why she cannot comply.

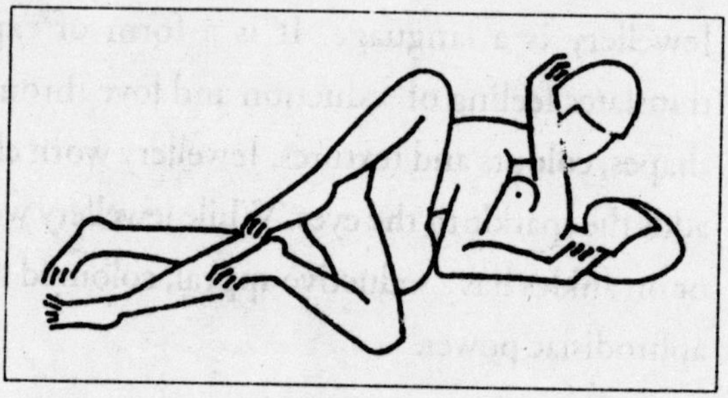

ANATOMY OF THE GENITAL ORGANS

The performance of the basic procreative function does not require any knowledge of anatomy. Even accomplished lovers don't need to know much about the structural details of sex organs. But some knowledge of sexual anatomy of genitals is helpful in understanding the sexual functions.

Are sex organs only a part of the reproductive system?

Sexual activity has been traditionally linked with procreation In lower animals this equation of sex with procreation is generally valid. As we developed further sexual activity became increasingly independent of reproduction. We can not procreate without sex, but we don't always engage in sex in order to procreate.

Many people think sex organs are dirty. There are men and

women who are married for years, have children but who have never looked frankly and searchingly at each other's genitals.

To many people the sex organs appear neither beautiful nor sexy when viewed directly, but reduce anxiety.

Should people look at their genitals?

Most people are ignorant about sexuality because they have a negative emotional attitude towards sex organs. People perceive their sexual anatomy as dirty and refrain from looking at it specially women. Even males, have negative feelings about sex organs. People should examine their and their partners genitals in a relaxed atmosphere.

(A) MALE GENITAL ORGANS

What are the external male genitals?

The external male sex organs consist of penis and hanging just below it is a small sac of skin called the scrotum containing a pair of testes.

What is the anatomy of a penis?

It is the male organ for copulation. It contains three parallel cylinders made of spongy tissue. Throngh one of which runs a tube i.e. urethra which conveys urine as well as semen.

Penis is a complex organ consisting externally of head or glans and a relatively long body or shaft. The glans is the most sensitive part having a large number of nerve endings. Separating the glans from the body of penis is a somewhat raised area known as the coronal ridge. The skin known as frenum connects the

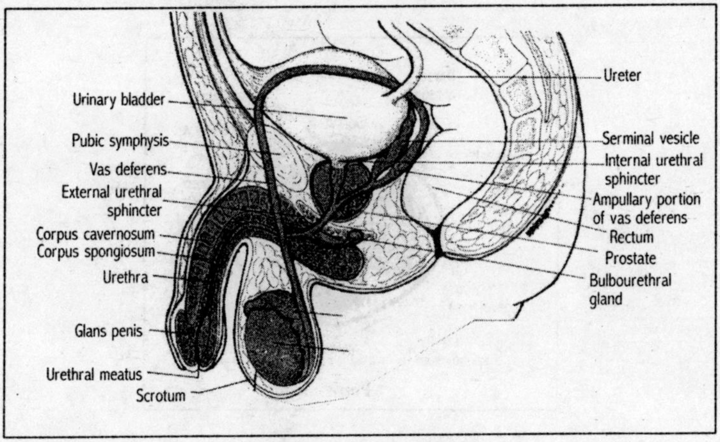

Male Reproductive Organs

glans and body. Corona and frenum both are sensitive to touch. The three cylinders of penis are structurally similar. Two of them are known as corpora cavernosa and the third is corpus spongiosum surrounding the urethra. Each cylinder is wrapped in a fibrous coat but cavernous bodies have an additional common wrapping which makes them a single structure. When flaccid these bodies cannot be seen but are easily felt when the penis is erect.

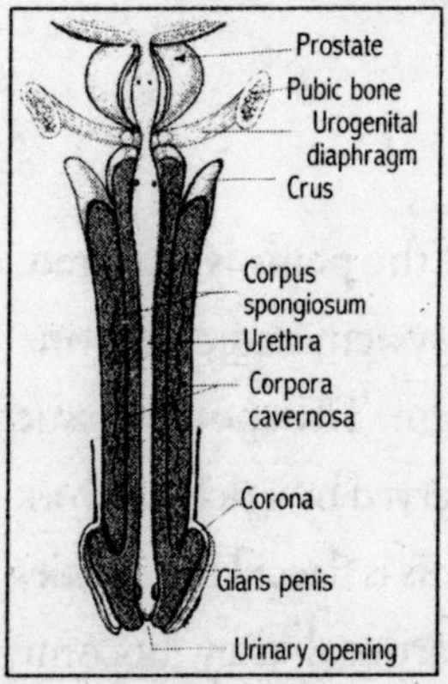

Penis

What about the skin over the penis?

The skin of the penis is arranged in loose folds allowing expansion during erection. When foreskin is present it gives a protection sheath over glans. In certain communities it is

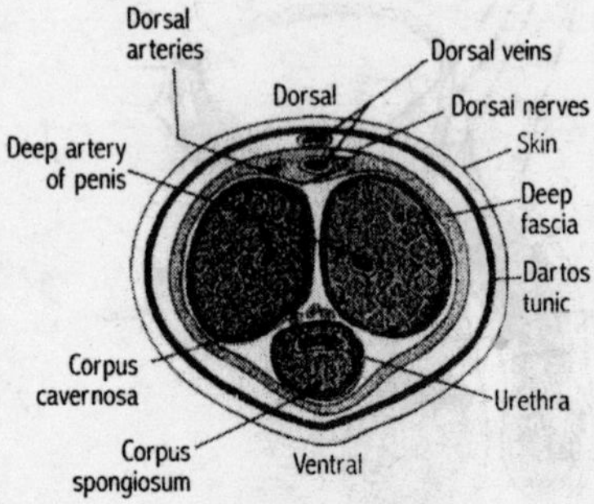

Penis

surgically cut known as circumcision. The advantage of circumcision is, that the whitish discharge smegma does not get any place to be collected. Smegma may give rise to the cancer of penis. In Muslims and Jews circumcision is performed as a symbolic religious rite.

How does erection take place?'

For entering into the vagina erection of the penis is required. All three factors blood supply, nervous system and endocrine system work together resulting in erection. The spongy tissue of the penis has irregular cavities and are served by a rich network of blood vessels and nerves. When the penis is flaccid the cavities contain little blood. During sexual arousal they become engorged and their constriction with in a tough fibrous coat results in stiffness.

What is glans penis?

The smooth rounded head of the penis is known as glans penis. It is formed by the free end of the spongy body which expands to shelter the tip of the cavernous bodies. The glans penis has a particular sexual importance. It is richly endowed with nerves and extremely sensitive. Most tactile stimulation of penis is transmitted through glans. The rest of the penis is less sensitive. Human penis has no bones.

What is scrotum?

Scrotum is a multilayered pouch. Its outer thin skin is darker in colour. It has many sweat glands and at puberty it develops a few hair.

Under it the muscle fibres are not under voluntary control but do contract due to cold and during excitement. When contracted it is heavily wrinkled.

What is the size of the penis?

The size of the penis is often a cause of curiosity and amusement as well as apprehension and concern. The average size of penis is 3 to 4 inches long when flaccid and some what 6 inches when erect. Its diameter is 1 1/4 inch and increases by 1/4 inch in erection.

Does a man's virility depend on the size of the penis?

No, not at all. Outer 1/3rd of vagina contains nerve fibres so even a 2 1/2 inches long penis is sufficient for successful sex. There is also no difference between circumcised and uncircumcised penises in sensitivity and excitability.

What do you understand by phallic worship?

Worship of male genitals is one of the oldest religious practice known. It is related to the fertility cults. In India Shiva, one of the three supreme gods is symbolically represented and worshipped as an erect penis.

What are internal sex organs?

These can be classified into functional units

Organs for the production of sperm-testes

System of ducts for storage and transport of sperm-epididymis, vas deferens, ejaculatory duct, urethra.

Delivery of sperm - penis.

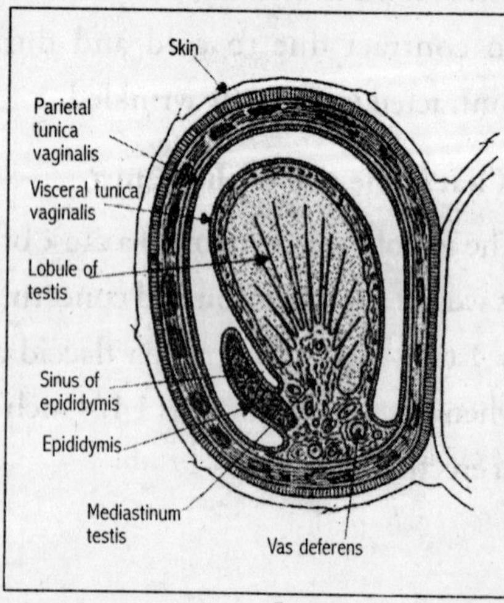

What is the anatomy of testes?

These produce sperm, as well as the male hormone testorterone. Two testicles are of same size 2x1x1 1/2 inches. Left one hangs lower down. Weight of testes is 28-30 gram. In old age these shrink.

What is the utility of seminiferous tubules?

Each lobe of testes is filled by seminiferous tubules. Each tubule is 1-3 feet long and the total length of all tubules measures several hundred yards. These tubules produce and store millions of sperms. Seminiferous tubules of newly born are solid cords. After puberty the tubules develop a hollow centre into which the sperms are released.

The second major function of the testes is to produce the male hormone.

Describe epididymis?

Each epididymis is a remarkably long tube, 20 feet long. It is twisted and convoluted. It is a C-shaped structure. At the end of epididymis is the vas deferens. It is a long tube that passes out of the scrotum and around the bladder to the prostate gland.

What is the role of the prostate?

It is the size and shape of a large chestnut consisting of three lobes.

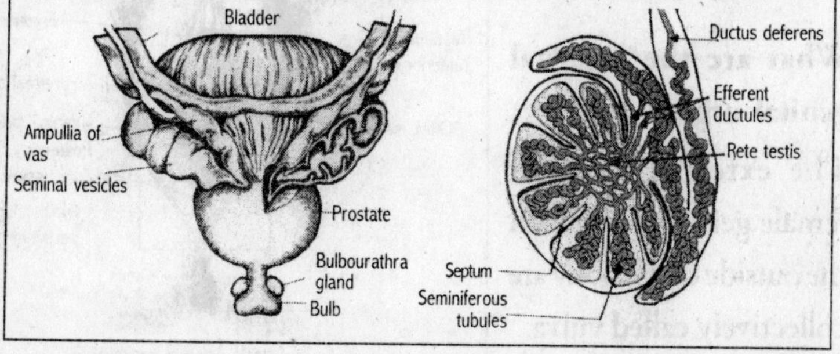

It produces seminal fluid and its characteristic odour. Prostate is small at birth, enlarges rapidly at puberty but usually shrinks in old age. When it becomes enlarged it interferes with urination.

What are seminal vesicles?

The seminal vesicles are two sacs each about 2 inches long. Each ends in a straight, narrow duct which joins the tip of vas deferens to form the ejaculatory duct. Each of these holds about 2-3 cubic centimeters of the fluid. These contribute fluids which initiates the mobility of sperm.

How does the Cowper's gland act?

These bulbo urethral glands are two pea sized structures flanking the penile urethra. These empty in urethra through a tiny duct. During sexual arousal these glands secrete a clear, sticky fluid that appears as a droplet at the tip of penis. It may result in coital lubricant. The fluid is alkaline and neutralizes the acidic urethra which may otherwise harm the sperm.

(B) FEMALE GENITAL ORGANS

What are the external genital organs?

The external parts of female genitals visible on the outside of the body are collectively called vulva.

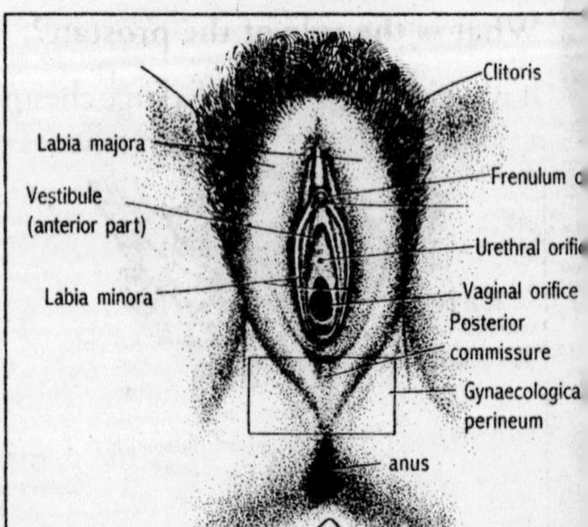

Female external genitalia

What is the mound of venus?

The most apparent part of the vulva is the most veneris which means the mound of venus. It is a fatty pad of tissue covered with pubic hair at the pubic bone in front of the body.

What is the role of vagina?

The physiological response of the vagina and penis to sexual stimulation are complementary. As the penis prepares for penetration the vagina prepares to recieve it.

How does vagina react during the excitement phase?

There develop 3 specific reactions

(i) expansion of the inner part

(ii) lubrication

(iii) change of colour

Moistening of the vaginal wall is the first sign of sexual response. Lubricatory function is of a clear and slippery vaginal fluid. This fluid is alkaline and tones down the acidity of the vagina.

What is the role of Bartholin glands?

Bartholin glands produce a discharge similar to Cowper's glands in a male. But it is scanty, erratic having lubricating value only.

How does the colour of vagina change?

Stretched walls of the vagina lose some of their normal wrinkled appearance. Due to increased blood supply the ordinary purple-red vaginal walls take on a darker hue.

What happens to the vagina during orgasm?

The area contracts rhythmically at an interval of 0.8 seconds from 3-15 times. After the first 3-6 contractions the movements become weaker and more widely spaced. This orgasmic pattern varies from person to person and in the same person from one orgasm to another.

How does clitoris play its role?

Clitoris is exclusively a sexual organ, but it does not play any role in reproduction and is independent of the urinary system. In sexual excitement the conjestion results in firmness of the clitoris.

It is highly sensitive. Practically all women perceive tactile stimulation in this area.

What are the responses of clitoris in the coital act?

During the excitement phase both the glans and shaft of the clitoris become congested. Glans of clitoris becomes double of its size.

During the plateau phase the entire clitoris is retracted under the clitoral hood and disappears from view.

During orgasm the clitoris remains hidden from view. Following an orgasm it quickly re-emerges from its retracted position. When orgasm has not occurred the engorgement of the glans and shaft of the clitoris may persist for hours and cause discomfort.

What are labia majora?

The labia majora are the outer lips of the vagina and are covered with pubic hair on their outer surfaces.

In nonpregnant females lips are flattened, thinner and more widely separated opening showing external genitals. During arousal congestion may be intense and labia remains swollen for several hours after all the sexual stimulation has ceased.

In ladies who have delivered children the majora are larger and more pendulous and may become permanently distended. Instead of flattening they become markedly engorged. Resolution is more rapid if orgasm occurs.

What is the role of minor lips?

Labia minor are inner lips, not having hair. These may fold over the vaginal opening. The inner lips contain extensive numbers of blood vessels and nerve endings. Direct stimulation to this area may be unpleasant but after sufficient arousal stimulation may be perceived as highly satisfying.

Do minor lips also change colour during sexual act?

During a plateau phase the minor lips become progressively pink or even bright red. In parou's woman the resulting colour is a more intense red or deeper wine colour.

In the resolution phase the swollen and discoloured minor lips return to normal.

What happens to the breasts during the erection phase?

Males also respond to sexual stimulation. Females respond better. It happens due to involuntary muscle fibres than vascular

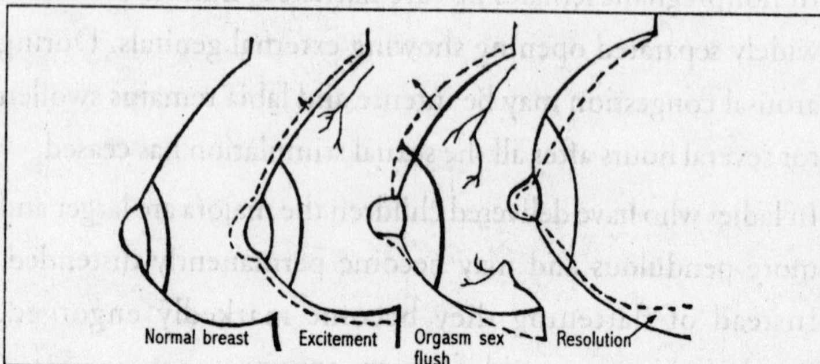

congestion. Enlargement of blood vessels is responsible for enlargement of breast as whole including areola.

How do breasts respond to the sexual act?

In the plateau phase the engorgement of areola is more marked. As a result nipples appear smaller. Breasts expands further. During orgasm the breasts show no further change. During resolution phase breasts return to normal size.

What changes in male breasts take place?

Changes in the male breasts are inconsistent and restricted to nipple erection. Male nipples are rarely stimulated directly.

Does skin colour also change during the sexual act?

Sexual activity results in a definite skin reaction, consisting of flushing, temperature change and perspiration.

What is flushing response?

The flushing response is more common in women. It appears as a discolouration like a rash in the lower chest. It then spreads to the breasts and rest of the chest and neck. In young girls the skin may become mottled. Sexual flush reaches its peak in the late plateau phase and disappears very quickly during resolution.

How does body temperature fluctuate during sex?

Although there is no evidence that the temperature of the body as a whole changes, people do frequently report feeling of warmth following orgasm. It may be due to superficial vasocongestion.

Perspiration occurs frequently during resolution phase. In man it may involve soles of feet and the palms of hand.

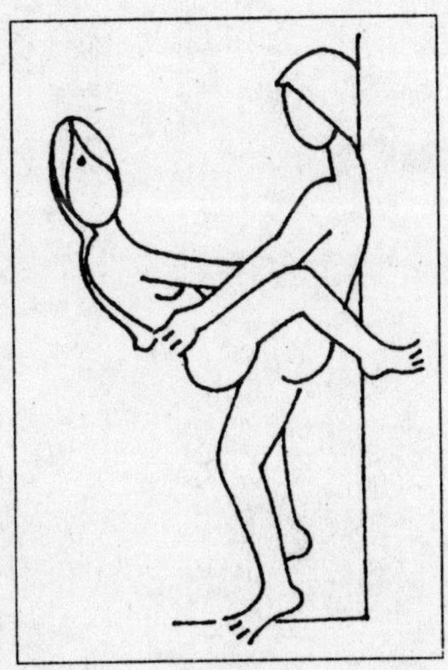

SEXUAL RESPONSE OF A WOMAN

What are different phases of the sexual response?

Sexual response has been divided into four phases

(i) Excitement or arousal phase

(ii) Plateau phase

(iii) Orgasm phase

(iv) Phase of resolution

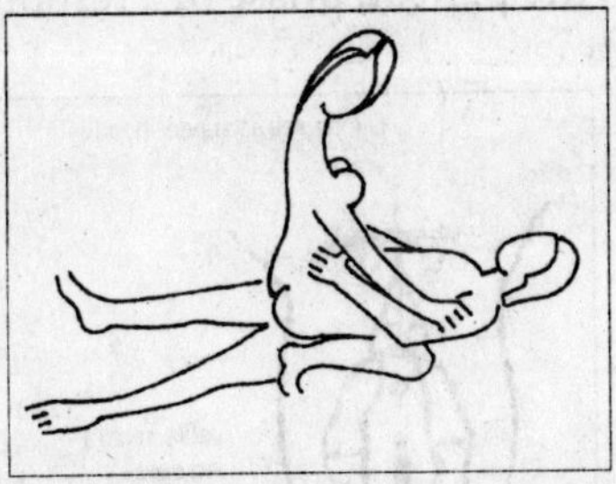

What happens in the excitement phase?

Most of the women have a heightened sexual interest often at midcycle or just before menstruation. Excitement phase of a woman tends to be slower in reaching its peak and last longer.

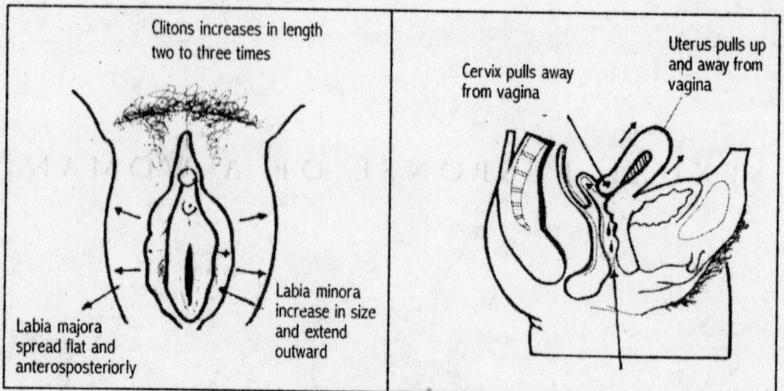

Excitement Phase

During it her nipples become erect and areola becomes swollen and dusky. Her clitoris increases in size. Lips around the vaginal entrance become softer and thicker.

Vagina becomes lubricated. Entrance becomes slippery to make coitus pain free.

What is the plateau phase?

There is no clear cut distinction between the excitement and the plateau phase of a response cycle. Blood pressure, pulse

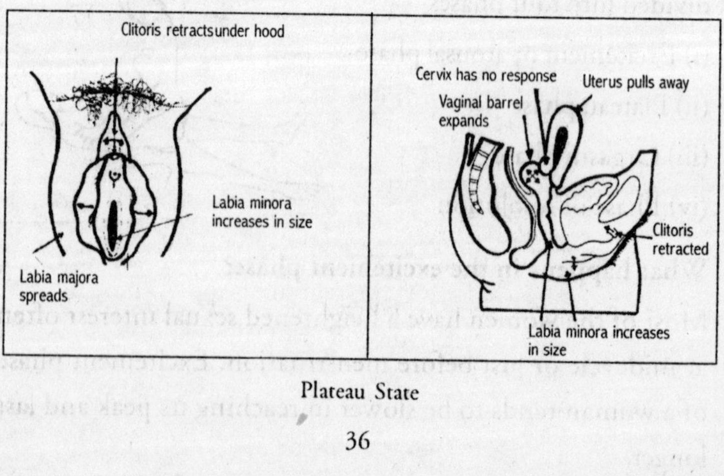

Plateau State

and breathing rates are maintained at a high level.

Myotonia may be seen in rigid muscles of the thigh and buttock. Some women make clawing and grasping movements.

Clitoris decreases in size and retracted so direct stimulation is not feasible.

Outer 1/3rd of vaginal engorgement reduces the diameter of the opening by about 30% so that vagina tightens around the male organ giving a satisfying pleasure.

Plateau phase is usually short in duration lasting for a few seconds. If one can prolong this phase it is more enjoyable.

What happens in the orgasmic phasse?

Orgasm is a feeling of intense pleasure which is the peak of

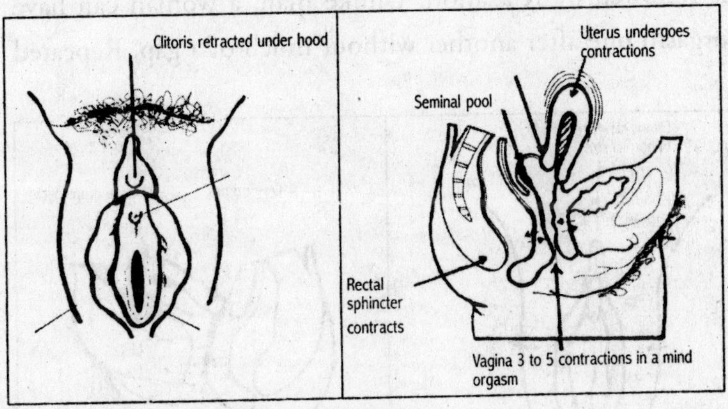

Orgasmic phase

sexual arousal. Feeling is intense pleasure which is deep in the pelvis and later spreads to the whole of body. There develop uncontrollable muscle movements a generalised tingling, a floating feeling, warmth and well being, a release of mental tension and exhilaration.

If she has inhibitions or develops the feeling that her man is 'using' her she may fail to attain orgasm.

Woman's orgasm is usually associated with some jerking thrusting movements of the thigh and pelvic muscles. The muscles of her womb and her vagina contract and some women have a more intense orgasm if she has erect penis deep inside the vagina so that she can rhythmically grip it by contracting vaginal muscles.

How does a woman feel during the resolution phase?

Convulsive muscle contractions and deep pleasure of orgasm is followed by relaxation. Unlike man, a woman can have orgasm one after another without much of a gap. Repeated

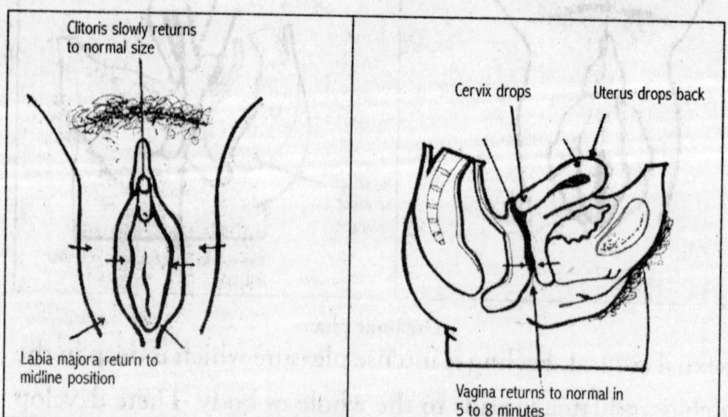

Resolution phase

stimulation and failure to achieve an orgasm may lead to physical and mental frustration. Repeated failure in attaining orgasm may lead to frustration.

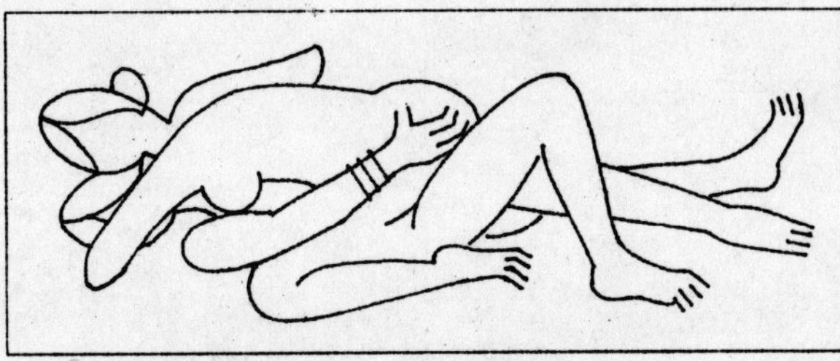

SEXUAL RESPONSE OF A MAN

What is the arousal phase in a man?

Love sets the mood and prepares the body for expressing the love through sexual intercourse.

During this period of growing excitement the penis becomes larger and more erect due to increased blood supply. Heart beat and blood pressure increase, breathing becomes heavier and nipples can grow erect. kissing, touching and caressing the genitals and other erogenous zones like lips, buttock are direct effective method of arousal.

What happens during the plateau phase?

During this phase the penis reaches its maximum size. The testicles increase by 50 percent and elevate to produce more forceful thrust in ejaculation. Sex flush develops in the upper half of the body.

If a man has been sexually excited for a fong time, the penis may secrete a few drops of seminal fluid before actual ejaculation. It may contain sperms and can make a woman pregnant.

What about the moments of orgasm in a Man?

Just before ejaculation a man develops a feeling of being about to come due to seminal fluid in urethral entrance. This feeling lasts for about four seconds and once the man feels that he cannot hold back orgasm he becomes verbal and produces sounds.

The penis ejaculates the sperm and seminal fluid about 1-3c.c. by rhythmic contractions. The more fluid will produce more pleasure. On two ejaculations a day the first ejaculation is more pleasurable because most fluid is ejaculated. Repeated orgasm will reduce the amount of seminal fluid ejaculated and it takes a few days to come to normal.

As regards coming together is concerned skilled lovers only can sometimes achieve simultaneous orgasm. Inexperienced partners rarely can manage it.

Love making can be satisfactory and fulfilling if one partner reaches a climax followed by another's.

What happens in the resolution phase?

During this phase the penis gradually loses its erection and returns to normal. A few people just after the discharge feels little tenderness in the penis. During this phase he does not tolerate his penis being fondled. The testicles return to their normal size and sex flux disappears.

After intercourse some men feel so tired that they go to sleep and are incapable of bringing their wives to orgasm even manually. They perspire a lot.

Once ejaculation takes place it takes long time to have an erection again. Refractory period goes on increasing as the age of person grows.

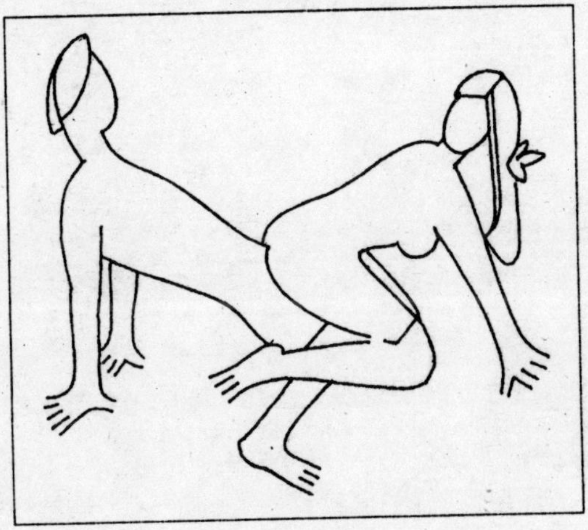

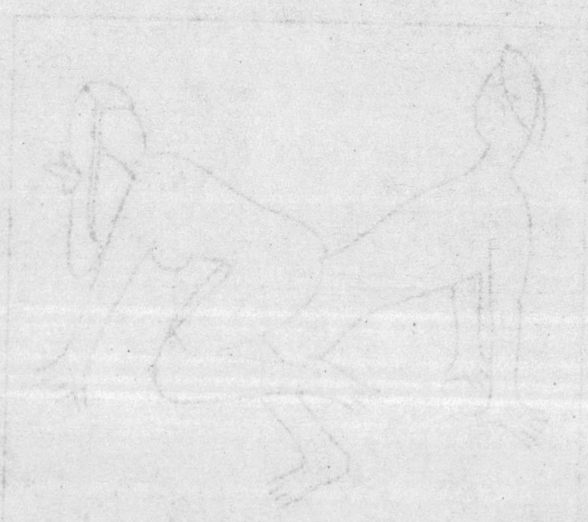

ADOLESCENCE

What do you understand by adolescence?

The period between childhood and puberty is adolescence extending from 10 to 19 years so. During this period only menstruation starts between the age of 10-16 years. Once menstruation starts a girl starts transforming into a woman.

What changes take place between girls during adolescence?

9-10 years. The bony pelvis begins to grow and attains a female shape.

Nipples bud.

- Fat begins to be deposited.

  11-13 years. Nipples increase in size

- Hair begins to appear on the pubis

- Internal and external genitals grow and develop
- The Vaginal wall thickens and vaginal secretions appear.

14-15 years. Breasts develops further and nipples become darker.

- Hair increases on the pubis and starts appearing on the arms pits.
- Acne appears

16-18 years. Increased fatty deposition occurs on hips and breasts.

- Periods become regular
- Growth of girls at 18 reahes at maximum.

What changes take place during adolescence in case of boys?

Puberty starts 2 years later in boys than girls.

- Penis, testicles and scrotum begin to enlarge
- Pubic hair increases. Hair develops over the upper lip and chin. The hair gradually becomes coarser and thicker.
- Larynx grows and causes the voice to deepen and break.
- Ejaculation begins when he is masturbating or fast asleep.
- Skin becomes oily and may develop acne.
- The armpits and genitals start smelling.

What psychological changes take place in girls during adolescence?

Personality changes in females develop due to physical changes and social pressure of parents to behave like a woman. Mixing with adult boys is restricted. Parents may not be able to accept that their children are growing into independent adults.

What is teenage sexuality?

Feeling about sex and sexuality begin to be formed in early childhood. At a young age children start getting pleasure from their bodies and it is influenced by parental attitude, education and social taboos.

They may start masturbating to relieve sex tension. Most adults continue masturbating when they don't get an opportunity of heterosexual sex.

Falling in love

It usually happens. If there is a relaxed relationship between parents and their daughter it becomes easier for them to discuss contraception and responsibilities of having an intercourse. A girl should know that she has to use a contraceptive to avoid an unwanted pregnancy.

Who becomes her guide?

In early adolescence her model is a female teacher or a relative. She obeys her, surrenders to her. This does not mean they are gay. Heterosexual attraction develops later on. Girls will find conflicting pressures being exerted on her.

What psychological changes take place in boys?

A boy's emotional and mental maturity may not be in tune with his physical appearance. He may look like an adult but behave like a child. Adolescent rebellion against figures of authority such as parents can be understood more easily when the gap between physical and social adulthood is realised.

When do boys develop their sexuality?

Even very young children get pleasure from their bodies. Their attitude towards sex depends not only on self discovery but also on the attitude and inhibitions of his parents and society. Unlike girls their sexual organs are easily visible and accessible and they play with their penis.

Many boys continue to spend most of their time with a group of friends of the same sex.Only when they approach their late teens they may start a serious relationship with girls.

What is the difference in the intensity of sexual desire between a boy and a girl?

A boy is sexually more aggressive and active while the female is receptive. Spontaneous arousal is not as frequent in girls as males.

What about the maturity of sex?

Scientists have declared that the man's sexual peak is around 19 and till 28 his physical capacity starts slipping down. According to them a woman reaches her peak at 32 and remains active till 38. It means in the present day context in India when boys peak and by the time they have their encounter on the honey moon night their decline has already begun while girls before reaching their peak already become a mother.

But there is another argument also that man may peak at 19 i.e. at this age he can indulge 3-4 times a day in sex. So it may simply be a physical act only, real enjoyment comes only after some experience, which cannot be at the age of 19 so we should not bother about the peak level but a maturity level which is far more important to make sex more fulfilling.

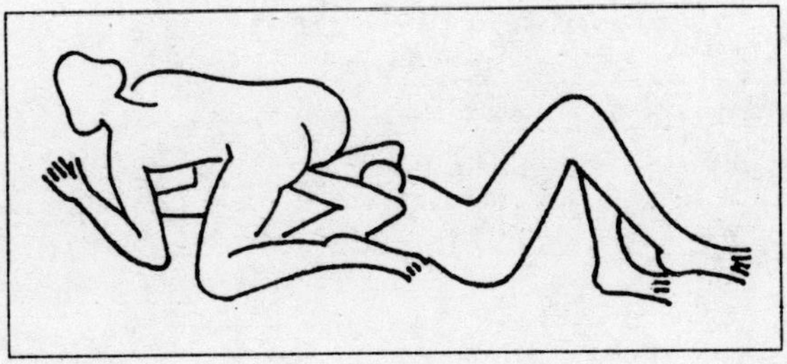

THE EFFECTS OF NAGGING

What is the role of nagging?

Most of the females don't realise that nagging is a weak expression of aggression. Only those females nag who have no self confidence. Nothing can destroy a partner's desire than nagging. There is a direct correlationship between nagging and inadequate relationship. Nagging can lead to sexual inhibition so sexual frustration can develop due to nagging.

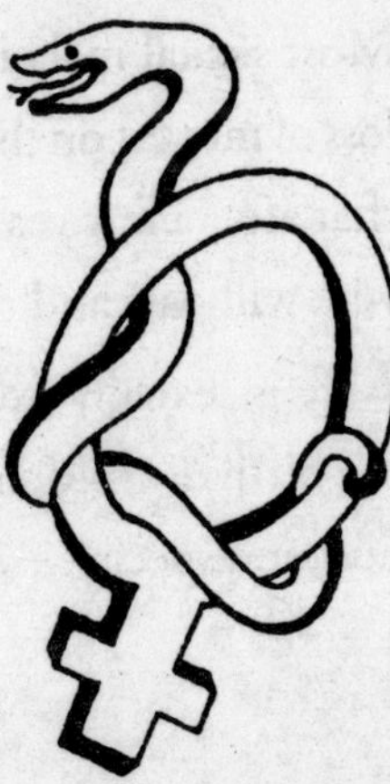

In what way do females nag?

If a female is sexually unsatisfied she should discuss the matter with her husband instead of nagging. It is expressed as 'No I am tired, I am having a headache, you are selfsh, you love me only in bed, you are sex crazy.' Some females prefer to remain busy in kitchen work, doing un-important work rather than giving company to the husband who is waiting in the bed room eagerly.

A woman who feels inadequate because she does not easily reach orgasm may nag her husband with complaints about his technique.

In which phase of life does nagging start?

Generally nagging starts after a couple has reached middle age. After many years of married life when she becomes dull, sex becomes routine and infrequent. After nagging a relationship generally looses its spontaneity and vigour. As joy and sexual satisfaction decrease petty irritation, grumbling and nagging grows. Wife's nagging mostly results in throwing her husband in the arms of other female.

Does nagging result in maladjustment in marriage?

Most sexual maladjustment in marriage seems to result from loss of interest on the part of either partner or both. It is assumed that after a few years of marriage the husband's interest in his wife will pale and the frequency of intercourse will drop.

Wife is sexually exciting for a few years after marriage. After the birth of children she starts losing interest in sex and in her husband specially.

SEXUAL MYTHS

Is masturbation unnatural?

The powerful sexual urge needs gratification during teenage. Media fuels the imagination-be it a film or book. Premarital sex still requires a lot of courage to break away from sanctioned behaviour and the only answer is masturbation. It is the form of sexual release easily available at any time with no fear of AIDS involved.

The fact is that masturbation is normal and does not render harm physically, mentally or sexually. However this fact is not digested by parents and teachers who fear that this practice will open gates to sexual promiscuity.

Can in any circumstance masturbation may prove unhealthy?

For some masturbation is resorted to release any kind of tension but some become so preoccupied with it that the ability to deal with a difficult situation ends up in masturbation. This may hamper the development of personality.

Wet dreams result in a loss of energy?

Involuntary ejaculation of semen which may have resulted from sexual excitement during a dream is called wet dream.

Adolescents are embarrassed by finding their undergarments wet and sticky in the morning after emission. Some fear it as a disease. It is not a 'swpandosh' Erection of penis during the night is a common phenomenon- a sort of nervous conditioned reflex. Erection can be seen even in a small baby. But when the semen starts forming in adolescence as the testes and other glands start functioning the erection is followed by emission naturally. It is a simple fact blown out of proportion. There is no question of losing one's potency.

Is bigger penis a source of better sex?

Adolescent boys tend to worry about the length of penis in its flaccid form. When alone they try to measure it with a scale and view it as a deficiency in growing up. The myth is that those with a short penis will not be able to provide complete sexual satisfaction to their partners or are less macho than their peers gifted with long ones. Some girls also think wrongly. On this the fact is that when erect all penises are the same. Actually only 1/3rd of vagina is sensitive to a touch sensation. The upper 2/3rd has a different sensation of pleasure. So length of the penis does not affect sexual pleasure. Erect penis may also deviate to one side.

Are bigger breasts more attractive to a man?

Human breast is the main target for erotic magazines. Bigger and conical breasts are sexually better is a myth, to look at and play with. Many girls wish to know how to improve the size so as to feel more feminine. Small and flat breasts give them an inferiority complex or make them a lesser woman. Bigger breasts are also not associated with a better quality lactation.

Is intact hymen indicative of virginity?

An intact hymen is indicative of virginity is a myth that has been passed down from one generation to another and cultures. Whether it started as a caution or to break premarital sex, is not known. Those girls who have had a sexual contact are afraid with guilt that their husbands on first night may discover that. Some women get plastic surgery done in the area of hymen so that they bleed on the first night.

Should coitus be done only during the night?

Most couples in our culture make love at night because it is convenient within the routine of every day life. But it is unwise always to relegate the coitus to the very last working moments of the day, because a certain amount of stamina and alertness are essential for real pleasure. It is advisable to change the time of coitus to the morning or middle of the day simply for variety. It gives a better chance of fertility too.

Is having sex without clothes an animal instinct?

Nudity during coitus is a subject of cultural and individual preferences. Men generally gets far more excitement from looking at female bodies than women do from looking at males. After some years of marriage women may also however prefer or love to be naked because it enhances intimacy. Full body comes in contact with each other.

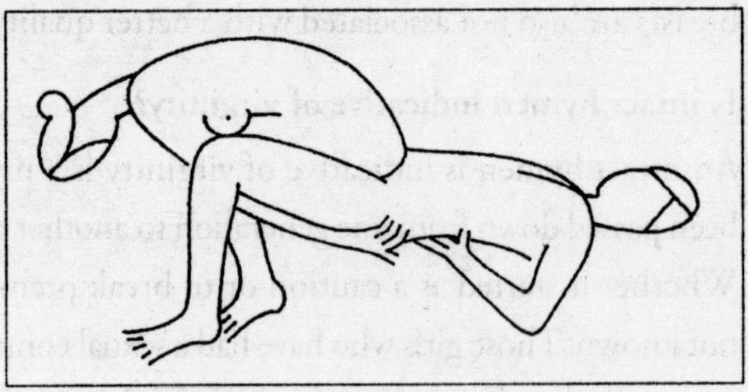

SEXUAL ADJUSTMENTS

What do modern husbands look for in their wives?

They don't want passive partners or inert recipients. They want responsive welcoming and often initiative lovers in their wives. They don't like the presence of guilt in their wives during change in positions while in bed.

What type of interpersonal love should be in marriage?

Interpersonal love invites the husband and wife to accept each other in toto without reservations, without differences. It recognises the fact that there are secrets beneath the protective layers of another's personality. It respects the qualities that make the marriage partner unique. Love is a fusion but without the loss of individuality.

Who should be the leader in love making?

Male has always been the leader in the sexual act but there is no reason why on some occasion a wife should not take initiative. Then the husband feels welcome and being wanted. The wife in making the advances has to shake off inhibitions. This increased fervour of hers stimulates her spouse still further.

Has the sexual role of man and woman changed?

Despite the new balance of power a husband still maintains the role of initiator and leader in foreplay. But women too have become more demanding in sex now and he has to attend to his wife's erotic needs and understanding her responses, as both draw pleasure out of it.

What should be the frequency of sex?

Frequency of intercourse is self regulatory and varies with an individual. Couples should have intercourse when they feel the desire and that is all. There is nothing like excess of sex.

What will happen if simultaneous desire is not there?

Sex desire is not necessarily always present in both partners at the same time and there is only one way to work out such time difference that is called adjustment. If a relationship is good it is seldom difficult for one to wait until the other's desire recurs. Impatience and over delay suggests that there is disharmony on misunderstanding in other areas of marriage.

What is the expectation of woman during sex?

It is in our culture for woman to be slug. For most Indian women sex is secondary and the technique does not matter much.

A woman admires a gentle and understanding male who makes her feel special as a woman, in bed and out of bed. She likes a man to be well mannered, kind and courteous.

What should a man know about a woman's sexuality?

For most women talking and feeling of being loved is more important than actual sex.

Husband should make time to talk during an evening walk or over a relaxed dinner. Husband should show his love which will pave the path for intimacy. A man should try to appreciate her skin, her dusky voice, her alluring lips, her captiviting eyes or her delightful smile. If she is little overweight she should not be criticized for that.

Does the woman like seriousness while making love?

Many people become too serious during love making. They forget to become romantically mischievous. Light heartedness can make intimate movements more relaxing. Lighter moments will sweep the pressure off the performance.

Can the husband tell when his wife is ready for coitus?

If husband and wife have become frank and there are no inhibitions then it is not difficult to sense each others reactions.

Physically there appears mucus secretions around the vulva from Bartholin glands. It makes penetration easier. It heightens sexual sensation also. Tension and anxiety during early marriage may reduce secretions.

How does personal hygiene affect sex environment?

Sex goes better if both have prepared their bodies before hand. Love making can be unpleasant because of poor hygiene.

Try to have a bath if you are going to make love. Make sure that your teeth and hair are clean. Your nails should be clean and cut.

Wash your genitals carefully so that you smell pleasant. Don't put strong deodorant which may mask the natural body odours.

How long should a sexual intercourse last?

It depends from couple to couple. Foreplay and after play may take any length of time but the period between intermission until orgasm in case of male may take 2 to 7 minutes while some men can prolong the coitus for 15-20 minutes.

Why girls generally don't talk about sex?

Certain girls may feel uncomfortable talking about sex or initiating any sexual activity because they have been raised to believe that good girls don't do these things.

In general a man has been encouraged to be more open. Some girls avoid being physically affectionate, because their husbands interpret it as a signal for readiness to have sex while they only wanted to be cuddled.

What is the image of a sexual male?

Man is urgent, aggressive, impatient, penetrating and ejaculating. The male still wrestles with his role seeking as a healthy husband to learn the lessons of tenderness and caring of sensitivity and sexuality in his lovemaking.

What is the image of a sexual female?

The biological picture of a sexual female describes her as passive, receptive, modest, retiring and submissive. She is supposed to be modest, conservative and passive. A male thinks that ladies are designed for motherhood first and for sexual pleasure later on.

How should a man behave during a woman's premenstrual tension phase?

For a considerable number of women premenstrual tension is a real and unpleasant phenomenon. The symptoms are irritability, depression and tiredness. A husband's understanding can be a great support during these unpleasant days. He should recognise that his wife's change of mood is the result of physical change over which she has no control.

He can arrange to give extra help in the house.

How should husband deal with a case of dyspareunia?

Painful intercourse is called dyspareunia. It is usually caused by physiological or anatomical disorders, irritation of the clitoris, infections and scarring of vagina, allergic reactions to birth control creams, jellies, diaphragms and tumors.

Psychological factors may also contribute to dyspareunia. Insufficient foreplay may result in lack of vaginal lubrication and tightening of vaginal musculature. The husband should give sufficient time in foreplay to get her ready.

How should a wife behave if the husband is involved in extramarital sex?

It is always healthy to maintain relations with only one man or woman as the case may be. Extramarital sex is a betrayal of trust in a love relationship. Still people become involved in extramarital sex due to deprivation of sexual activity, illness or sexual dysfunction at home. Most extramarital affair reflects what is missing in the marriage. Wife who is in the habit of nagging i.e. refusing sex on some pretext or another pushes her husband for extramarital sex. A woman should be ready to break monotony in sex by adopting different postures & initiating sex on occasions. How so ever beautiful the wife may be the husband gets bored with same sex and the same positions. There should be enrichment of some kind.

How to react to a masturbating husband?

Yes, increased rate of masturbation amongst married persons may act as compensation for frustration in marital coitus, unwilling and non cooperative wife. Otherwise also masturbation is not a sin. If the wife co-operates and adjusts with the urgent needs of husband masturbation may be avoided.

Why some females masturbate to orgasm?

Some young girls masturbate when other forms of sexual pleasure are missing because they don't have a boy friend or don't want to be exploited by them.

Many married woman masturbate when the husband is not able to reach them to orgasm. Congestion of the satisfied pelvic organs takes a long time to come to normal and the process is painful. A man should learn to delay his ejaculation, give sufficient time in foreplay to satisfy the women. Some ladies masturbate when they are sad, lonely or under stress using it as a last resort and getting it over to have a sound sleep.

Is there any difference between orgasm during intercourse and masturbation?

Orgasm during masturbation is intense. One is free to reach orgasm as he or she wants. One need not to regulate his pleasure with the pleasure of his sex partner.

How to react if the husband wants to have sex during menses?

It is quite possible to make love during periods. Some women feel sexy during their periods. Even with the tampon on one can have sex. During this period woman remains well lubricated. There is no harm.

Does spontaneous sex bring a change?

Yes but some couples are never spontaneous and many make love on a fixed, regular basis on the same night of week, each week, but quick sex is great.

Indeed some women have orgasm only with quickie sex. They like to be taken hard and fast. This proves to them that they are so desirable that the husband cannot help him self wanting them. This proves highly flattering to their femaleness.

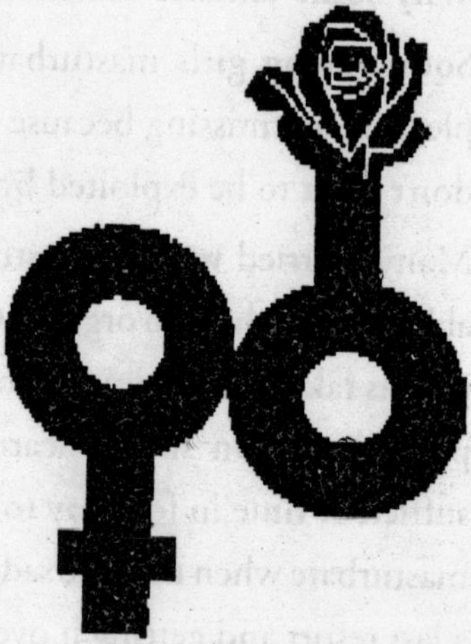

If you expect that spontaneous sex is on cards wear a loose nighty without a bra because the layer of clothes with multiple buttons are nothing but a nuisance in the heat of the moment.

Should wife suggest an experiment of making love?

Why not? Routine approach leads to routine sex, predictable and boring. Sex is taken as granted with few demands in return. Many women fall into a sexual rut because of the fear that they will be misunderstood and will be unacceptable to the partner. To suggest something which sounds perverted or odd exposes to her being rejected, even ridiculed. They fear that suggesting something unusual might put their partner off depriving them of sex.

Is after play necessary for women?

Orgasm is not the end of sex play. Most men after the discharge turn to the side and go to sleep. For them the game is over. But after love making the husband should kiss and caress her. Tell her how much you want and care for her. Make it obvious that it is her pleasure you are seeking.

Is oral sex dirty?

No, not at all. Good sex takes place more in mind then anywhere else. There are two ways for a couple to use oral sex. They can use it as a foreplay before penetration or can use it as an alternative form of intercourse. Whichever way a couple uses it, oral sex can provide exquisite sensations not only for the recipient but also for the giver.

Many women believe and feel that the genital area is dirty and the act is some what unpleasant for them.

How to deal with an impotent husband?

Impotent man is one who cannot achieve or maintain erection sufficiently for intercourse. The man suffering from impotence is frustrated, anxious and depressed. He feels humiliated by his repeated failures in front of his partner. His confidence in his manliness is shattered. If it is psychogenic the woman can reassure the husband and get him investigated and treated.

1. after play necessary for women

Orgasm [illegible] [illegible] sex [illegible] than [illegible] the [illegible] [illegible] to the side and [illegible] [illegible]. For them the game [illegible]. [illegible] making the husband [illegible] and [illegible] [illegible] [illegible] [illegible] [illegible].

[illegible] [illegible]

[illegible] [illegible] [illegible] take place [illegible] Whether [illegible] [illegible] [illegible] [illegible] [illegible] [illegible] [illegible] [illegible] [illegible] [illegible]

Many women [illegible] and [illegible] [illegible] [illegible] [illegible] [illegible] [illegible]

How to deal with an impotent husband

[illegible]

[illegible] [illegible] [illegible] [illegible] [illegible] [illegible] [illegible] [illegible] [illegible] [illegible] [illegible]

[illegible] [illegible] [illegible] [illegible]

FAMILY PLANNING

Why family planning?

The birth of the first child is an event of incomparable joy to parents. The child becomes the centre of their lives. Mothers shower all their love, attention and care on new born. The husband is naturally deprived of this exclusive attention and the care of his beloved wife. Hence proper spacing of 2-3 years after marriage is suggested if it is not a late marriage.

A young husband can plan his fatherhood. Family planning enables him not to be overburdened with the problem of home and service.

What factors help in taking the decision on the use of a specific contraceptive?

Sexual activity just after marriage contributes to unwanted

pregnancy. Condom is best for man to use but withdrawl requires considerable control. For females it can be pills but pills may not prove useful from the day of bridal night. It has to be regulated from the date of menstruation.

What is condom?

It is the most widely available contraceptive. It is a thin sheet placed over glans and shaft of penis acting as a physical barrier. It prevents pregnancy by blocking the passage of semen and is reliable when used from start to finish. A sheath worn over penis can be traced back as far as 1350 BC.

What are the advantages of a condom?

- Condom allows the husband to participate actively in contraception.
- It is easily available and at a low cost
- Condom allows men to maintain their erection longer and prevent premature ejaculation.
- There is no post coital leakage of semen from vagina spoiling aesthetics.
- It protects from sexually transmitted disease.
- Lubricated condoms can reduce mechanical friction and irritation of penis or vagina increasing sexual pleasure.

What are the disadvantages of condom?

- 'Unacceptable to some men and women because of lack of genital contact reducing women's enjoyment.

'Sexual intercourse has to be interrupted and the condom had to be put on after erection.

- 'It can be torn by finger nails or may slip while taking out spilling the semen.

What are combination pills?

For a period of 21 days a dose of female hormones oestrogen and progesteron is taken in the form of small tablets.

The first course of tablets should be started latest by the 5th day of menstrual cycle counting the first day of bleeding as Ist day. This should be started by taking the first pill from the packet marked as start till the full packet is finished.

New pack should be started the very next day by taking the first tablet from the packet marked as start.

If the user forgets to take the pill for a day it should be taken immediately and then continued as usual. Pills can be used for 3-5 years.

What are the undesirable side effects of pills?

Side effects include nausea and vomiting, dizziness, headache, heaviness in breast and weight gain. There may be break through bleeding.

What is copper T?

It is an intrauterine device. The presence of copper exerts a potent antifertility effect. The safest and best time for insertion of copper 'T' is when menstruation stops. It is inserted in the woman's uterus by a trained ANM. The whole procedure takes a few minutes.

It may result in cramping in the abdomen for first few days. There may develop vaginal discharge or irregular menses for first few months.

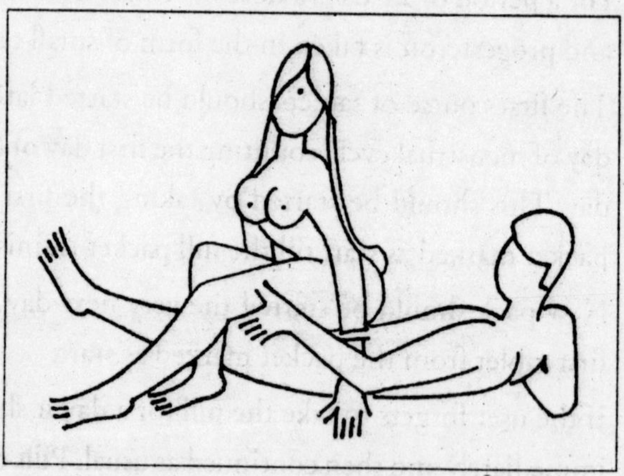

SEXUAL POSITIONS

Old Indian books describe as many as 84 positions. Some positions ensure more effective stimulation of genital, bringing a woman to orgasm while others make mutual care easier. Some require atheletic stamina while others are useful in pregnancy.

What is face to face position?

It is a woman with her back, her knees slightly drawn up and the man lving above her. In this position the couple can kiss

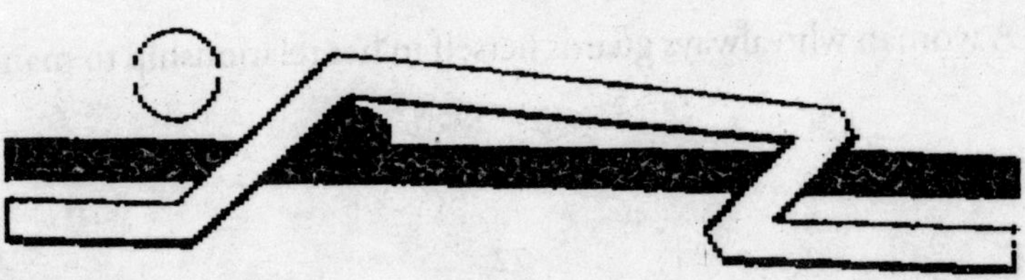

easily, play with the breasts and respond to each others facial expressions while their bodies are in close contact. She can caress her partner as she wishes. Man can control his movements and thrust deeply.

How does the woman on top helps?

In this position the woman lies above the man. It is useful when a man is tired and his hands are free to play with breasts but the man's pelvic thrusts remain limited and difficult to synchronise with that of a woman's movements. Making love in different surroundings and at unaccostomed times can itself provide stimulation and excitement. There can be fullest penetration and due to stimulation of clitoris she can be brought to orgasm.

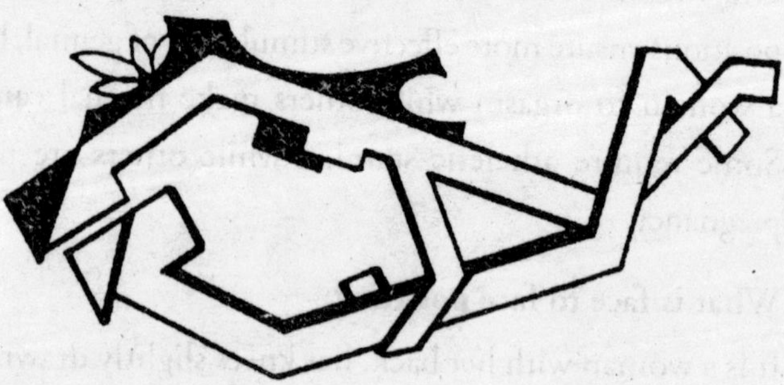

What is rear entery position?

A woman who always guards herself in her relationship to man is the one who prefers rear entery position. She states that she does not like the missionary position because it makes her feel "being pinned down" although in rear entery she is surrendering more control to man but she does not have to face him directly. In this position she remains greatly excited and her entire body twitches during orgasm.

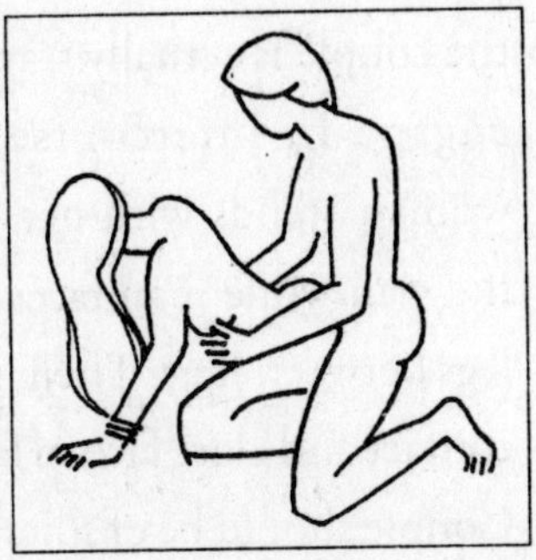

Rear Entery

What type of men generally prefer rear entery?

Men who prefer the rear entery position usually like to be in the sexual pattern. Often they want to keep maximum emotional distance from woman.

What is side by side position?

In this each partner lifes on one side facing the other. It is least common but is most democratic in this position movements may be restricted. So it becomes necessary that the couple be equally involved in thrusting toward one another. Partners are face to face. Each has a free hand with which to caress the other's back and buttocks.

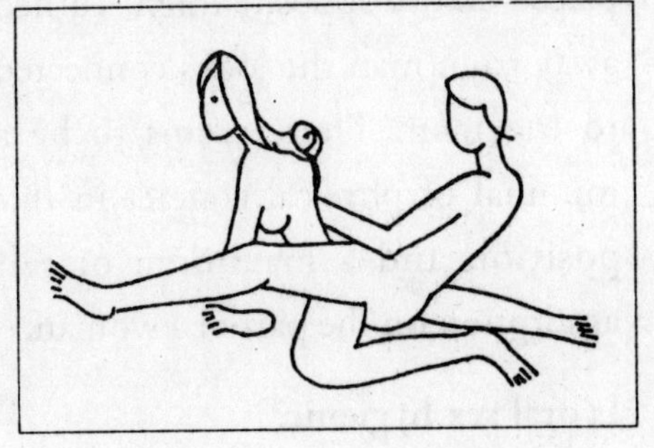

What about sex in standing position?

The use of legs takes on a different kind of significance when the couple is actually standing as they engage in intercourse. Generally woman stands with her back against the wall while man faces her with his legs between hers. There is much skin contact and close face to face intimacy. Couple should be of suitable height to thurst each other.

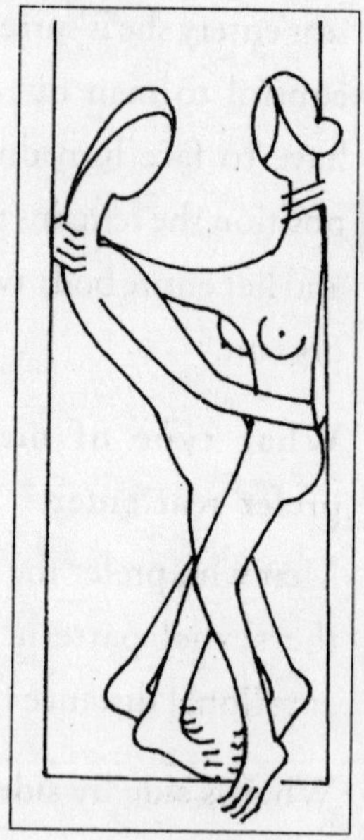

What do you understand by lotus position?

In the lotus position man his supine while the woman sits on toy of him. Her back is turned to his face folding her legs into classic oriental position of contemplation with each foot placed on the opposite thigh. Turned away from man she looks connected to the man. There seems to be a minimal of physical contact in this position and a maximum of self absorption on the part of a woman.

Is oral sex hygienic?

Oral sex the use of mouth as another

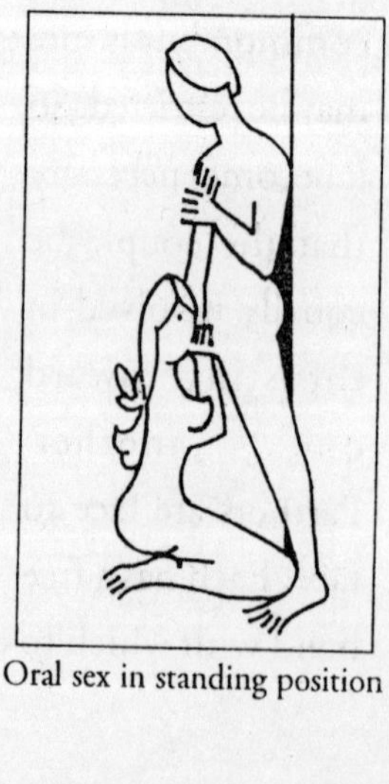

Oral sex in standing position

entery port is becoming more openly acknowledged. Although less flexible than hand mouth is capable of broader range of activities. Tongue creates a number of different sensations. It can stroke, lick and nip or kiss. There are wide variety of using oral sex. If genitals are properly washed and cleaned there may not be any hitch.

Can one enjoy 69 position?

If both partners are willing and ready to enjoy each other's genitals orally, it can be a very satisfying experience. This way both can attain orgasm.

What do you understand by anal sex?

When man enters in anus instead of her vagina. And mucus membrane is very thin and can give way out. Passage of anal canal is little angular.

How masturbation helps in coitus?

Masturbatory techniques are used during arousal phase leading on to subsequent intercourse and mutual orgasm, it can be very helpful in bringing both partners to the same level of excitement.

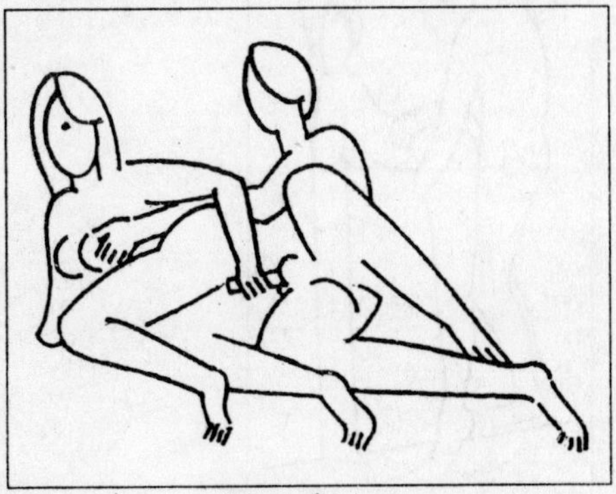

Masturbation

The masturbation of one partner alone often occurs after the other has achieved orgasm through intercourse.

Thus a man who loses his erection after ejaculation may use his fingers to help the woman to achieve an orgasm.

Will change of place/spot for sex will add the pleasure of sex?

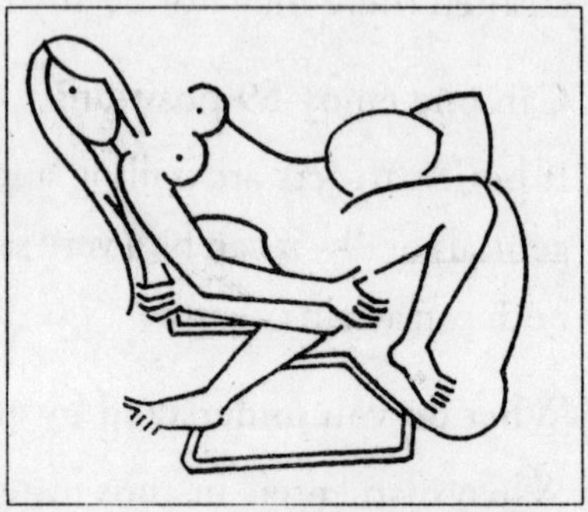

Yes it will break the monotony. For this purpose other than bed, sofa, rolling chair, 'S' shaped chair can be used comfortably.

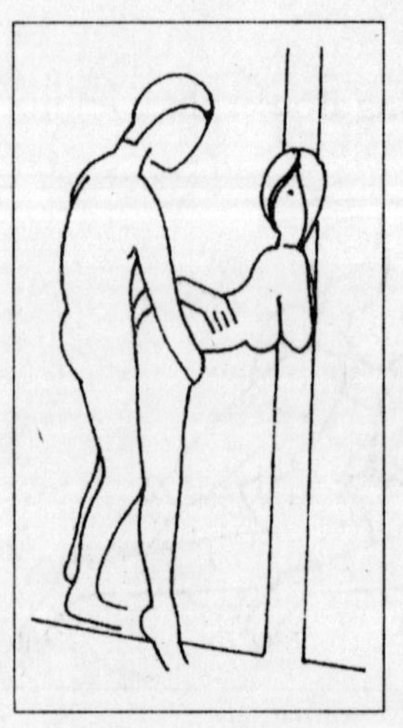

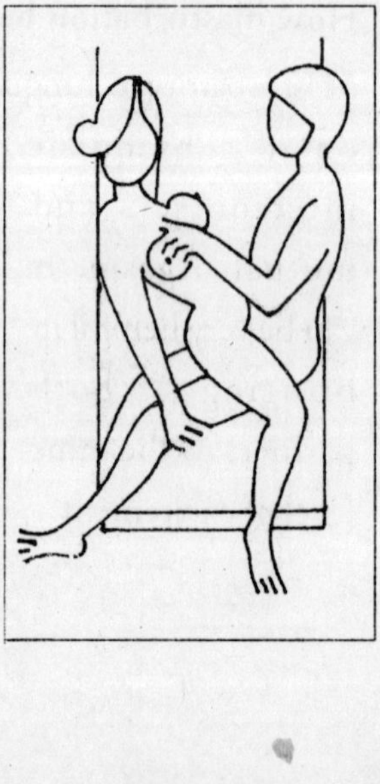

Joy of Marriage

Joy of Marriage

L C Gupta, M.D., D.Sc
Abhishek Gupta M.D. DRM

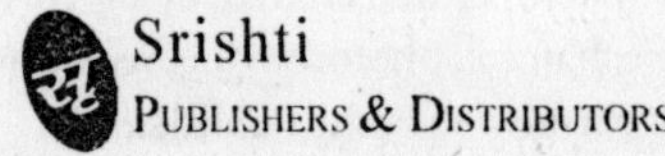

Srishti
PUBLISHERS & DISTRIBUTORS

Srishti Publishers & Distributors
64-A, Adhchini
Sri Aurobindo Marg
New Delhi 110 017
srishtipublishers@forindia.com
srishtipublishers@yahoo.com

First published by Srishti Publishers & Distributors in 2003

ISBN 81-88575-16-x

Typeset in AGaramond 11pt. by Skumar at Srishti

PREFACE

Marriage is undoubtedly good for individuals. Society looks upon marriage as a mechanism for controlling sexual behaviour. It is a v5ery effective device for lifelong fidelity to one partner. The perceptions of men and woman differ, owing to changes marriage brings in their respective lives.

To make marriage a success a woman makes concessions, submissions, and also changes her level of expectations. The woman truly reshapes herself for her husband and for in-laws

A successful working woman is also a wife and a mother and hence the pressure of performance for her on all fronts is tremendous. A supportive family can ease her burden by the sharing of responsibilities.

L.C. Gupta

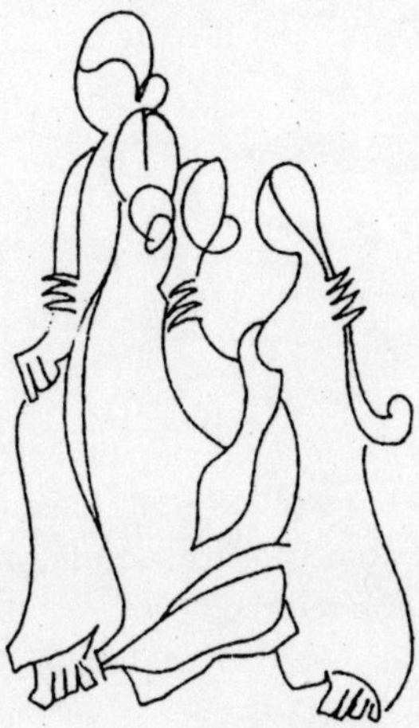

CONTENTS

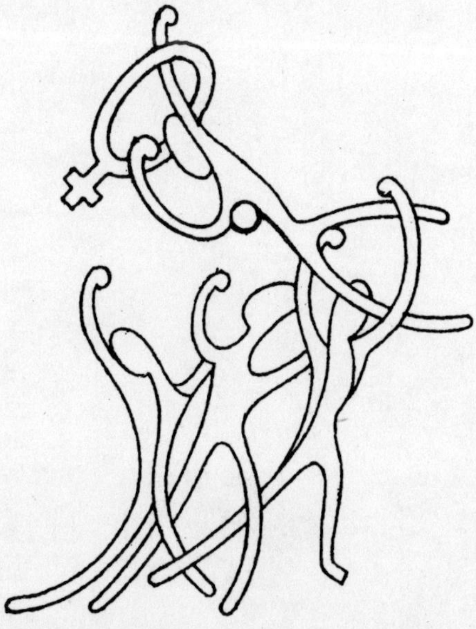

FAMILY

The year 1994 which was declared the International year of the family by United Nations drew our attention to that basic unit of society which we tend to take for granted. Family whether it consists of a single couple with children or many couples related to each other is absolutely essential for human development. It provides the necessary physical, social and emotional growth for an individual and forms a link between different sections of society keeping it together.

The institution of marriage and the event of child bearing are considered essential for family life. Every individual has a right to marry. It is with in this charmed circle that he gets the necessary growth to go out and serve the society and make a life for himself to the best of his ability.

There are natural human and caring qualities in a family relationship, wherein a child gets physical and mental security and stability. Hence the need to strengthen the tie of family is essential for any society which believes in progress and development. It is also necessary to protect the rights of individuals within the family and family it self within the society.

In present times some may say that the word family is losing its significance. In India we are moving from joint families to a nuclear family stressing more and more on individual development which sometimes might clash with the interests of the family as a whole. In the west there are couples living together without marriage, the single parent families without children are becoming more popular. The hectic pace of living in modern societies is responsible for this to some extent. Also there are certain problems concerned with family like violence against the women, inequality among different family members, lesbianism and bigamy and matters concerning money which might be responsible for the disintegration in the family in the present day society.

Advantages

Inspite of all these problems a strong family system is a must for any developed society. For the basic growth of an individual a strong and a happy family is essential. It is here that one learns to share and care. In the process of growing up a child imbibes all that he needs to learn regarding social and cultural heritage. Inside his family a child develops a strong sense of identity and belonging.

Since family is a micro unit of a society or a nation, for the well being of a nation too it is necessary to have a strong family. In the absence of that we will have individuals who are insecure, isolated, selfish and prone to more violence. According to experts children born out of wedlock or those of broken homes are non productive. The reluctance to commit oneself to family ties ultimately leads to a meaningless existence.

In India we have always had a strong family system. The tradition of having a joint family is also something which we can be proud of. Although these days we come across more of nuclear families which may be due to compulsion instead of choice. The growing materialistic attitude is also a major factor in the disintegration of a family. Lack of tolerance and the desire to be free from family ties can also be noted amongst present generation.

Yet the solution to all these problems mainly lies in our need to have a strong and united family which has a broad leucrative set up.

Gradually people are realizing the significance of having a joint family which lays its foundation on love and sacrifice. A nuclear family may be more popular now a days because of the fast pace of our life yet a return of the joint family system is what we need in the present circumstances. Joint family teaches lessons in love, obedience, tolerance and imparts a sense of sharing and belonging to its members. Even in a nuclear familiar family the head has to put in an effort to help the family together. The lesson of love has to be taught with in the family itself.

MARRIAGE

Marriage is an institution that regulates the relationship between a man and a woman for the creation of a family.

Marriage is the history of society itself. The evolutionary theory indicates that primeval practice was group marriage based on the sharing of partners and children within a group ignorant of their paternity. Later on this gave way to a matrilineal system and ultimately to a patrichal one.

Polygamy has been an outcome of the advent of the patrichal system. More wives and many children formed part of the property of a man.

The common methods of marriage were

- marriage by consent
- marriage by purchase

- marriage by service
- marriage by force

2. Purpose of marriage

In older times marriage was regarded as a private matter and could easily be dissolved. Manu considered marriage as a social institution for regulation of proper relations between the two sexes. The aim of Hindu marriage is said to be **dharma** (duty) **Praja** (progeny) and **rati** (pleasure) Fulfilment of religious duty was the main aim of marriage. Man needed a wife mainly for the fulfilment of religious duty. Hence on the death of a wife the man therefore was obliged to remarry immediately. For a woman marriage was considered the aim of her life. It was considered impossible for her to gain 'moksha' until she was married. There are instances where old spinsters were married before or after death so that their soul could go to heaven. The second aim of marriage was perpetuation of family. Getting a male child was important. During marriage ceremony the groom tells the bride "I am heaven and you are earth. Come let us join together so that we may generate a male child, a son for the sake of increasing the wealth." Infertility was next to widowhood. A husband had the social sanction of remarriage if the wife could not become pregnant.

3. Kinds of Marriage

Rituals: Prabhu described eight forms of marriage. Brahma form, Daiva form, the Arsha form and Prajapatya form where the maiden is given as a gift by the father or guardian to the bridegroom. The remaining four forms of marriage have no merits because Asura form involves price for the bride, the Gandharva form does not involve the family, the Raksha form is marriage by force and Paishacha form is marriage by fraud. In early vedic period the process of marriage consisted of the bridegroom's taking the hand of the bride and offerings were made to Agni. Gods were invoked to give their blessings to the newly married couples to give them health and wealth. Mantras were uttered to drive away evil spirits.

Marital relationship

In a marital relationship the husband and wife were bound to each other till death. In the first four categories divorce was not possible but in the last four couples could dissolve it by consent.

Females were taught the lesson of Pativarta i.e. devotion to the husband.

Manu said that the husband is to be worshipped even if he is not good.

Vedas indicate that polygamy is natural, where as polyandry where a woman has more than one husband is unnatural.

Love and marriage

Love can last but a lot of investment is needed to keep love alive in a marriage. In a marriage both the partners have to try, one partner cannot go on loving if the other is indifferent.

Love is an emotion not only physical but spiritual as well. Physical intimacy is extremely important in keeping a marriage intact. Being wrapped in their career people don't have sufficient time for it. Love lasts when you want to make it last, what is required to keep the love alive is mutual understanding of the two persons involved with each other. Both should be prepared to 'give' from time to time. They must spend time together and lot of it at home. Small body gestures of intimacy are as important as the act of love. With thoughtful little gestures both must create gestures in their life for each other.

Women in the coming times will be more complex and different than the women of today. The wife has ceased to be only the home maker, instead she has become an enterpreneur herself. She is also developing other areas of interest outside the home.

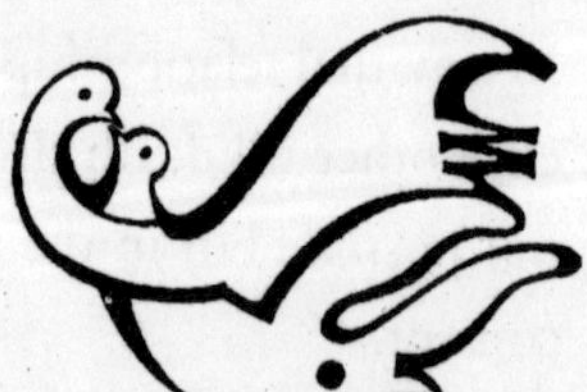

Sacred Space

Who Understands Love?

Happiness, sadness, knowledge, and love

lived on an island.
One day the island began to sink. So all
the feelings prepared
their boats to leave.

*

Love stayed. She wanted to preserve the island
paradise until the last
possible moment. When the island was almost
under, love decided it
was time to leave. She needed help. Richness
was passing by in a
grand boat. Love asked: "Richness, can I come
with you on your boat?"
Richness answered: "I'm sorry, but there is a
lot of silver and gold on
my boat – there would be no room for you."

*

The Love saw Vanity in a beautiful vessel.
She cried out for help.
"I can't help you", Vanity said, "You are
all wet and will damage
my beautiful boat."

*

Next, Love pleaded with Sadness: "Please let me
go with you." But Sadness
declined, saying he needed to be alone.
Then, Love saw Happiness.
Love cried out, "Happiness, please take
me with you." But Happiness
was so overjoyed that he didn't hear
Love calling to him.

*

Love began to cry. Then, she heard a voice:
"Come Love, I will take
you with me." It was an elder. Love felt so
blessed and overjoyed
that she forgot to ask the elder his name.
When they arrived on
land the elder went on his way. Love realised.
How much she owed
the elder.

*

Love then found Knowledge and asked, "Who
helped me?" "It was
Time," Knowledge answered. "Only Time is
capable of understanding how great Love is."

Unknown Poet

Marriage for ever

- Spend quality time together. There must not be grumbling sessions specially during love making. Finger pointing is detrimental.
- Never take each other for granted. One should express appreciation even after sex.
- Never compare your spouse to anyone else.
- Romance can start with a cup of tea if it is prepared by the husband.
- Wife should avoid nagging. She should not say 'I am not in the mood' or 'I am having a headache' or 'you are only interested in sex.' Sex is a better way to relax.
- Always appreciate each other all the time, cheat in games, splash water and have a bath together.
- Have soft teasing and keep touching each other.
- Romance is not about being with each other all the time, but it is about communication. Giving pleasure to each other.
- Remember you are never too busy to love.

Importance of sex for a happy marriage.

Ninety percent of couples have a less than perfect sexual relationship. There are many women who have never experienced an orgasm but are leading a happy life. It means performance is not as important as the feelings they bring or fail to bring to their sexual relationship. Many women are more interested in closeness than in a simple orgasm. Only when the husband fails to hold her in his arms a woman feels empty, rejected and being used.

Failure to connect is only one kind of sexual difficulty that may spoil marriage. Most couples find that their sexual encounters are influenced by job pressures, financial worries and fatigue. Woman's inability to relax can be the cause of problem in their sex lives. For them it is not possible to adjust to instant intimacy once the doors of the bed room are closed.

If you are keen to revitalise your sexual relationship, better communication both physical as well as emotional are critical. It is the quantity and quality of sexual relations that makes or breaks a marriage. Try to define for yourself and for your spouse your complaints and pleasures. Many couples are uncomfortable and shy in making specific requests. Open talks and experiments are vital. Feed back is required for other partner's pleasure.

How a man treats his wife out of bed greatly influences her response in bed. Harsh words, inattentiveness and criticism can make it difficult for a woman to be an enthusiastic lover. Women see everything in their life as inter connected while a man tends to be compartmentalised. For a woman affection and sexuality cannot be compartmentalised. For her good sex is a continuation of closeness and affection. Women want romance, cuddling, hand holding and kissing out of bed room. Your marriage is the most important relationship in your life. Finding time to be together should be a top priority. It is not only to make love but to express that you love each other in words as well through gestures.

Making a marriage successful

When two persons marry they expect to have a better life. Worst moments of your life ruin a relationship. Hard times can bring a husband and wife closer or tear their relationship apart. At the time of trouble it is easier to undermine your marriage. To avoid this one should restrain the urge to blame the spouse for wrong happenings. For such people marriage provides an easy available scape goat. Actually in marriage there is no way to win against your own spouse. Either you both win or both lose. During rough time feeling of being loved gives you strength. At such time of crisis body language is more eloquent than words. Husbands very often don't want to discuss the plus and minus points of their marriage critically.

Before putting pressure on your spouse to talk about his feelings and instead of interpreting silence as indifference one should remember that talking may be more difficult but sensible.

Develop flexibility in emotions. In a healthy marriage partners are to express their positive feelings when circumstances are adverse.

Being a wife and mother

The job of a housewife can be compared to the exhilaration of living with a man, loving him and helping him to hum and sing with children.

A wife should take pride in the strength and the achievements of her husband, analyse his areas of weakness and also encounter his uncertainties. Respecting your man's job is very important because when you marry a person you marry his job too. Doing a job perfectly gives man a pleasure just as motherhood does it to a woman.

Wife should learn the basic act of giving without demanding. Unsuccessful wives demand love and affection with no return. Most men desperately need a support against which to test ideas, hopes and inner conflicts which they cannot resolve alone. They need a loving wife in whom they confide their inner most thoughts and feelings without the fear of being ridiculed or rejected. There may be occasions where a wife has to hold her tongue to avoid arguments. Let him know that you need him in bed and equally otherwise too. Use your talents. Marriage need not limit your horizons. If you have a talent for photography, interior decoration or writing poems don't let it gather dust. Use it to improve yourself and your family. With the mother in law don't make an issue over small things. Don't be alarmed if you and your husband differ on some matter. Marriage is an inseparable partnership.

Kids or no kids

Number of couples are refusing to use children as a domestic cement. I see a daughter trustingly holding dady's index finger in the advertisement but I don't feel the need to push a pram myself' says Rita.

Today a few Indians have started following the trend of NO KIDS-NO COMPULSION. Married couples are deciding not to reproduce themselves. Earlier society was dependent on each other but now a days every thing is available in the market and can be purchased. Dependency has ceased.

Considering the population explosion and modernity a woman is no longer morally bound to pay her debt to nature, not bound to breed any more. Now they don't want to go to temples to pray for a child. Couples who want to have a free life don't want to have children.

But childless females don't develop that affection. Nature initiates the maternal instinct only during post pregnancy period when the offspring is on the breast. Human infants require prolonged care unlike animals.

Endless quest of the childless woman

Womanhood is not complete without being a proud mother of a child more so in the Indian content. The childless woman particularly a poor woman can face staggering social and economic pressures. She is often abused of being barren even when the problem may lie with her husband. She may be threatened with desertion or be asked to tolerate her husband's second marriage. She has no guaranteed access to proper infertility treatment. Her choices are ill equipped hospitals with a careless staff or a jungle of fertility specialists who are ready to snatch her money. When unable to seek medical help she goes to faith healers where she may even be sexually abused. Educated class tries to adopt a child of a known relative from the very beginning. Adopting an orphan child carries a risk of unknown parenthood because the child will inherit genes from his parents only and his I.Q., behaviour all depends on it only, the only plus point is that such child will not leave you while a relative's child can look forward to break away from such a relationship, when he or she becomes adult.

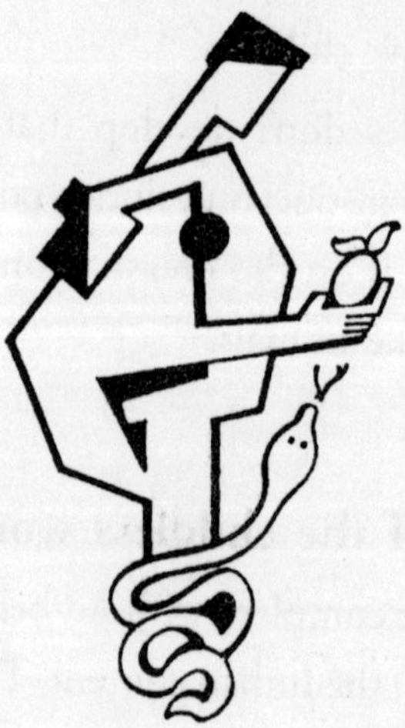

MOTHERHOOD

It is well known that only a mother is able to look after her child well. Even if something goes wrong with the child's education and behaviour the father always puts the blame on the mother. It is also true that children of working women may not be able to enjoy the mother's love, affection and guidance in full.

In todays busy and competitive world mother hood may bring isolation, confusion and insecurity to some women. Such women may not be sentimentally attached to the child as it used to be in the past.

Every individual varies in her attitude of motherhood and her capacity to handle it. There is nothing like a good and bad mother. Different approaches to motherhood depend on a woman's stamina and temperament whether they feed the baby on time or change his diaper as soon as it is soiled. Some will feel an instant love for their child at birth others may even be frightened. Some women realise that being a mother is one of the most thrilling experiences and the greatest privilege while some describe it as exhaustion, the boredom they experience in bringing up small children.

In Indian society women primarily are seen as mothers and those who don't want to become mothers are noted as perverse and deviant.

Most of the new inexperienced mothers belong to nuclear families while girls who come from joint families develop an experience of bringing up children. This familiarity helps when it comes to bring up her own babies.

For most parents birth of the first child seems to be a major psychological turning point. Every parent desires to give the child a better life and greater happiness than they had as a child.

Bonding between Woman

In the West more women will be living together in the next decade. For the Indian society female bonding is nothing new. In a traditional joint family where girls are not permitted to go out of the house to make friends they always prefer friendship, comfort, companionship and soul mates in their bhabhi, aunty and cousins.

When a husband remains out for long the woman finds herself turning to another woman. They sympathise with each other and provide each other with emotional anchors. In some cases mature empathy may stop short of intimacy scaring to cross the line.

In India social norms have always forced women to stick together. Lack of co-education, strict parents and social taboos ensure that men and women can hardly be friends. Since the girls are encouraged from the beginning to help in household chores, it inevitably leads them to being in company of other females more than males.

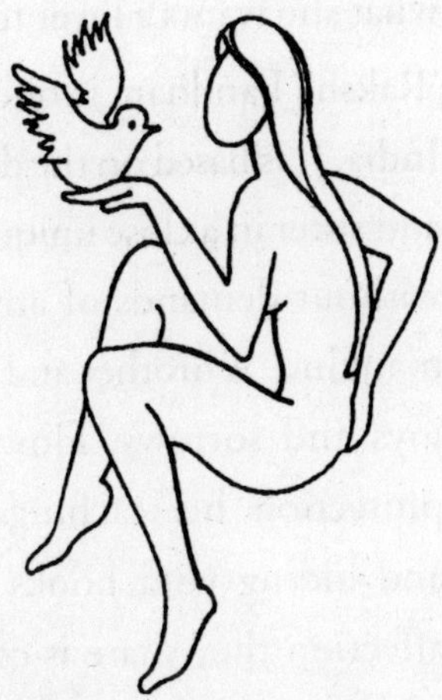

Brothers and Sisters

A brother is a confidante in sister's life. A brother offers a perspective on the tangled emotions and his gentle teasing is a blessed antidote to the parents admonishments. Brothers of a younger age group can be a good company. Good bhabhi finds a younger brother in the form of a 'dewar' He protects her from the unwanted company of the opposite sex. Younger brothers often bring out the motherly feelings in a sister. She looks after her like a son and prepares herself for future motherhood.

The discovery of a reflection of her own emotions in her brother/dewar is a gift of reassurance when a girl feels blue. To a bhabhi her dewar's love is a perfect valentine. Perfect because he loves his sister/sister in law for her essence which is exactly what she wants a lover to recognise.

'Raksha bandhan' is one of the most sentimental festivals of India. It is based on the deep emotional ties that bind a brother and sister in a close unique bond, the sacred relationship of life without demands of any type that nature has bestowed on mankind. A brother and sister grow up together, share similar joys and sorrows. How one can forget an elder brother's protection, his teachings or younger brother's frank remarks and hiding your books and letters. The bond of love and affection they share is complete which cannot be compared with any relationship. To symbolise this profound relationship the sister ties a rakhi on the right hand wrist of all her brothers and applies teeka on their forehead. With the tying of this string she bestows deep affection and blessings on her brother and wishes them joy and prosperity while the brother promises to protect her from all odds in her life.

Once a girl has tied rakhi to some boy at any cost they cannot marry in future. Society does not allow to break the moral bond. Boys who are not having any sister sometimes select some girl and regard her as sister and get the rakhi tied. She gets the honour of his sister in the family.

Husband and wife both should respect and honour such a relationship.

WOMAN HAS NOTHING TO DO TO ATTRACT A MAN. THE FACT THAT SHE IS A WOMAN IS SUFFICIENT.

ACTUALLY THERE IS NO MORE BEUTIFUL A WOMAN THAN IN LOVE.

MOTHER IN LAW

A mother-in-law and daughter-in-law can seldom live harmoniously. Many daughters-in-laws complain -'she sits on our head like a presiding deity' the jealous watch dog of her son, the bearer of house keys and the last word on all family matters.

Actually when a lady becomes a mother-in-law she is in the menopausal phase when she feels irritated and, full of frustration. She is likely to suffer from depression. Hormonal changes have spoiled her personality. At this juncture daughter in law enters the family and it becomes very difficult for a possessive mother in law to give their son to another woman. More over a new comer becomes an easy prey for her.

The traditional adversary can be turned into a friend with a little patience, a little tact and just a little healthy selfishness.

Many daughters-in-laws do live with mothers- in-law happily. They bring home a good movie, a packed dinner and spend a cosy evening, laughing together. They enjoy eating together, playing cards and teasing each other.

Psychologists say that unspoken fears can make a mother-in-law feel very vulnerable which could manifest in suspicion and hostility towards the young daughter-in-law. Many mother-in-law will not allow the young bride to enter the kitchen. She will insist on looking after all her son's needs, even packing his lunch to office. Daughter-in-law is bound to feel like a stranger, left out of an intimate mother son relationship. But if the daughter-in-law keeps patience and tries to be near and dear of her it could bridge the distance. If you give her importance, consult her and take due guidance in preparing the food she will stop treating you as a trespasser.

Even if she strikes out of jealousy, in time to come and in response to your soft behaviour she will come to terms, adjust and get on with you. If you resist the temptation to react, she will eventually find a 'daughter' in you.

Most in law relationships have some measure of formality in them. Pushed too far, formality can turn into resentment. What most mothers-in-law expect is that you should jump out of bed early in the morning and prepare tea for her and give her with respect. Touching of feet works as a three inch motor and you will get a tight hug in return.

Some of the acrimonious conflicts arise when the son's wife does not fit the expected image that her mother in law has been unconsciously nurturing for years. Then a cold war could ensue which could manifest as either verbal withdrawl or subtle rejection. You cannot change your mother in law but you can stay calm. It is always better to hold cold silence than a hot war.

You have to trust your mother in law. Don't keep your cupboards locked and jewellery hidden from her. This secrecy can hurt the old woman very badly.

On the contrary even simply sharing the news and happenings in your life can help bring warmth in your relationship. Laughing together can change the mood of a relationship. Ask her to tell you about her son's childhood. Look through the photo albums together. Appreciate the mother-in-law in the old photos. Once you stop playing a tug of war over your husband you may discover that you actually like each other. Keep your mother in law in high spirit.

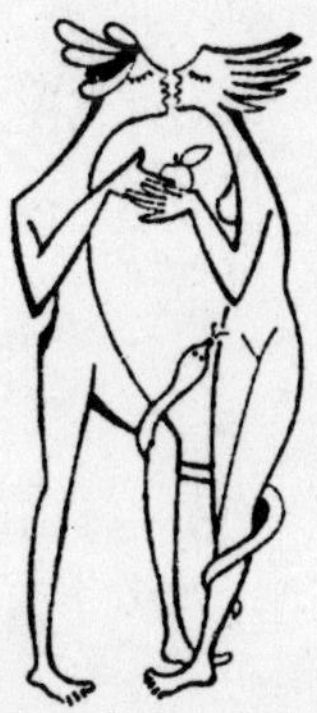

A WORKING WOMAN

In India ladies go to work not out of choice but due to compulsions. Married women and single mothers are subject to a much greater strain than married men. A woman working alone in a primarily male organization may be subject to more stress. She is put under psychological pressure. She is seen as an outsider and one who is different from others.

Married working women have to perform the duties of a house wife too. They have to prepare the children for school, clean the house, do shopping, cook meals, supervise children doing their home work, attend school functions, care for each member of the family and ailing parents in law and manage to do work at office and uphold the position successfully.

Majority of women work because they have to and want to.

They do because one salary today is rarely sufficient to keep up a family's standard.

Women as Managers and Leaders

It is believed that women handle stress better than men when both are exposed to the same trauma. But a woman who is at the middle management level is exposed to harassment and plays a considerable price in terms of menstrual problem, dysmenorrhoea and miscarriages. Women have a right of choice of equal opportunity with the advent of oral contraceptives and freedom from unplanned pregnancies.

Many females may be natural leaders and good managers and may ascend to managerial and supervisory roles. But on occasions they have to pay a high cost to rise to the top. With promotion females may be transferred to other locations and such movements may prove traumatic. Moving children from one school to another hampers their standard of education. Secondly family life is disturbed because if the husband is not in service then he may not have a chance to be transferred along with his wife.

Very often a female may find it difficult to be happy in a man's job. Women are psychologically and sociologically inclined to be conciliatory and nurturing. This sort of a soft woman while she makes an excellent supervision may not be entirely happy in a leadership role which calls for certain aggressive, assertive and musculine qualities.

There are women graduating every day in different professions specially medical, law, MBA and the future is very bright for them but progress up the professional ladder may cost a great deal in terms of anxiety, tension and illness. Sometimes tiredness, boredom due to a monotonus job and role burden, take their toll in the form of both physical and mental exhaustion.

Thirty years back most of the working women were single but now most of them are married. For doing a job financial motives are important and most of the women make the decision to work so that she may raise the living standard of the family. Secondly she works to over come loneliness and boredom once children have become independent.

Working Women and Early Motherhood

Today the pattern of work for most women is to work till marriage. Once she become a young mother she leaves the job and again tries to work when the children have become independent. During this period part time work can fit in with the needs of their children and the members of the family. Working women without training are not able to cope with the demands of the family and of the work place.

Many women go out to work because of an intellectual need. They find at home frustration and inferiority. If a woman has worked some time in she past the will always like to join again when her responsibilities are over.

Pressures on a Working Woman

On being interviewed many of the mothers admitted the feeling of guilt for leaving their children alone. But being divorced, widowed or being a single parent, they have to take up a job due to financial compulsions.

In lucid moments guilt does seems to be a non affordable luxury. Whatever be the life style of a woman but to her children she has a priority over her husband. Otherwise also children need a caring adult and for that grand parents are a good help to children. As long as they are well cared for in the absence of mother they may not suffer intellectually, emotionally or mentally.

A woman who is to persue her career actively and is keen to succeed to get promotion has to devote a lot of energy for that and in the process she is left with minimal energy to look after her children. The husband may feel neglected.

In the natural course women don't have the tendency to act selfishly. Biologically they put their children and their mates before themselves. But the paradox is that a successful working woman has to put herself on many occasions, higher on her list of priorities than her natural inclinations.

If you want to climb the ladder you have to be selfish about your desires perhaps more selfish than you would like to be. As a working mother it becomes difficult to please all the members of family.

Double-income families

Historically women have always been active workers along side of their men supporting the family economy directly or indirectly. But so far the females work contribution was largely confined to the unorganized sector such as agriculture or home based production. Job participation of women has resulted in the rise of double income families. Actually urbanisation and the rising costs have burdened the earning of the sole earner. Educational services are the largest single avenue of employment for women in urban as well as rural areas, otherwise concentration is in the traditional, low paid, less prestigious jobs. Women are mainly employed as nurses, and as health technicians, clerks, stenotypists and telephone operators.

It is true that income of the family increases but ladies are pulled between extended familial duties and obligations of their job requirement. Moreover it is noticed that a woman's higher status of work place does not change her status at home, although she starts taking part in decision making. Participating more in domestic affairs but on occasions even husband develops jealousy.

Sexual harassment

There are sections of women who are sexually harassed by their bosses and have no one to help. Explicitly, touching and discussing intimate sexual incidents at the work place are common offensive forms of sexual harassment. Repeated invitation to date, forcing to stay late night in the office and giving her a lift home after having tea at a hotel are common practices applied by seniors. About 10 percent of women experience physical contact, verbal overtures & loud comments. Fear of the loss of job, hostility at work and social stigma prevent the woman from complaining about it.

Almost any one can be a victim of sexual harassment. Job hierarchy often determines vulnerability. It is more severe for women working in unorganised sectors where jobs are not secured. Here are some tips to avoid sexual harassment.

- Tell the harasser to simply stop and state clearly that his attentions are unwanted.
- Talk to some one near and dear in your office about such a harassment so that either he may tell the harasser or become a witness.
- Informally raise the issue at work and find out if any other colleague has had similar experiences at work place.

Legislations to protect common worker

It is better to know various legislations protecting the women workers

- Equal remuneration act 1976 which seeks to provide equal pay for equal work irrespective of gender.
- Maternity benefit act 1961 gives to all workers the right to protect their health, before during and after pregnancy.
- Factories act 1948 besides providing for a safe hygienic work place workers to provide for the establishment of creches or day care centres if the factory employees include more than 30 women.
- Laws on sexual harassment. According to revised rule on rape the affected woman's statement may be taken as a sufficient proof against the colleagues.

A Corporate wife

The high ranking, well compensated life styles of hi flyers are formed by powerful, cultural, legal and economic forces. It looks glamourous but the corporate ladder is a steep one. There may be a big car, membership to exclusive clubs, handful of servants, large houses filled with all the gadgets that money can buy, but at the end of the day life can turn out to be lonely and empty.

Loneliness of the corporate wife is due to two reasons

- husband is hardly ever in town.
- back stabbing of the corporate world.

Most of the husbands flag off the day at 6.30 in the morning and the day ends at night with a dinner engagement. Keeping pace with the husband's career and demands of family responsibilities may result in depression.

Some women may be very ambitious enjoying the heady power of success and money. Through the blue smoky haze at parties she may shrug off her tiredness and paste a smile on her face to attract and please bosses.

In modern time a husband requires a co-operative wife to reach the top and here are some useful tips to such a wife

- Keep your channels of communications open with the boss and his wife off and on.
- Do small favours for the boss. Offer to locate Ayahas, teachers and cooks.
- Be always well dressed, striking enough to attract attention of the person concerned. But never out do the big man's wife.
- Whenever you enter a party meet the top guys and their wives first. Stick to them and laugh when they desire.
- Check with your husband whom he considers part of his team. Be gracious to them for your husband's needs.

- Always appear unruffled and capable despite children's examination or other arrangements.

Be friendly to the secretary of the boss by giving presents. She can give you valuable information.

Improve your communication skill to be retained.

- Think clearly and have a clear idea of what you want to write/tell.
- Have a clear articulation of thoughts.
- Have a good knowledge of language and its grammar.
- Improve knowledge of your subject. The quality of content is important. Wide reading will ensure vast knowledge.
- Catch the attention of the target audience and be poised.
- Listen, retain and express. Listen when you are spoken to, retain what you have heard and express at the right time.

Listening and retaining are as important as talking. What you learn is by listening and what you express is by retaining.

WIFE BEATING

Wife beating is a crime of rage and power. It is a means of exercising control. The male dominates after making her afraid. In India it is prevalent in the lower class. The batterer feels that he has a right to the extent of duty to control his wife.

Wife battering has been going on for centuries. Only durning the last few decades it has been banned in certain countries. But even now the police does not interfere thinking that it is a private matter. Typically husbands blame their partner for the violence. Still why women don't leave him? The answer may differ in different cases. Some battered women may be loving their husband. Some try to ignore violence. Some don't leave because they don't have confidence and have no choice except to live with him.

The battered women often feel trapped. Violence often starts with a push or slap. If no one interferes it may go worse. Alcoholic husbands generally indulge in wife beating, when specially she requests him not to drink. The more he beats, more he drinks. Children of such families are sufferers.

Another cause may be not getting sufficient dowry in marriage. Husbands along with in laws either beat or burn the bride. Under the new law punishment up to 6 years if something bad happens like this husband and in laws may be presumed guilty and punished. Under another amendment if woman's husband or in laws torture her mentally or physically may be jailed for 3 years.

But by and large battered wife does not get sympathy in our society. Police also takes action when she is seriously injured. Due to marriage being something scared victim's parents also remain reluctant to take any stern action and advice her to go back to husband. No body wants to give a shelter to a battered wife.

Religious faith of a woman

Throughout the world girls are more religious than boys. Manu formed so many religious and social guide lines to curb sexuality and liberty.

There was a time when the formal practice of any religion was old fashioned but today the perception is changing fast. The young boys have even started attending religious prayers. Now they go to temples and pray either for passing the examination, getting desired wife or a job. Difficulties in life and frustrations have made them more religious. The number of young girls trying to renew their ties with faith is increasing.

After marriage if the woman is not able to conceive, she becomes a regular visitor of religious places. Persons of one religion are visiting worship places of other religion. Lots of Hindus go to Ajmer Sharif.

In a world where survival is tough and competition is keen where relationships are fragile and institutions like marriage and family are suffering in the form of sickness, financial set backs and emotional upheavals, religion becomes the source of strength.

Kusum has my faith in religion as it helps escape the overall stress that permeates every aspect of our existence.

Women believe more and more that there is an invisible force in nature who guides and protects their children and husband. An Indian woman observes fast for the welfare of her husband and also to protect children's interest.

Revivalism is in because many feel disillusioned in institutions and find themselves incapable of addressing their needs and aspirations. Religion does provide a sense of security both spiritual and material. Frustration and disillusionment are responsible for returning to an organised faith. When life and society don't provide you with desired environment, religion comes handy.

LEADERSHIP

Perhaps much has been written and less agreed upon regarding leadership. Leadership is a word on everyone's lips. The young attack it and the old grow wistful for it. Experts claim it and scholars want it. Politicians wish they did and pretend it. Thus it is very difficult to define leadership. Leadership is a vision accompanied with the ability to translate that vision into reality. There is a vast difference between management and leadership. To manage means to bring about, to accomplish, to have charge of or responsibility for conduct. Leading is influencing, guiding in direction, course, action and opinion. The distinction is crucial. Managers are people who do the right things. Leadership consists in marshalling the skills possessed by a majority but used by a minority. Managers become leaders when they learn to take a stand to take risks, to anticipate, initiate and innovate. Leadership skills were once thought to be a matter of birth. Leaders were supposed to be born and not made but in the present context this theory has been rejected. It is presumed that some kind of leadership opportunity is available to practically every one. How best to utilize this opportunity is to develop leadership.

In most places present day leadership is a directive leadership. It creates a situation in which the subordinates tend to feel dependant upon the leader. A successful leader is the conductor of an orchestra rather than a one man band.

Marital Breakdown

Sociological research shows that marriages have a greater chance of success when both partners are from the same social, ethnic and racial back ground with similar religious and moral beliefs. When there are common needs and expectations, there is a greater likelihood of marital success.

Visible breakdown

- Divorce
- Separation

Masked breakdown

- One partner is unhappy
- Both partners are unhappy

Statistics of divorce in society is a significant yet a limited indicator. It is not possible to find out an evidence of a masked breakdown. A couple may go on drag living together because of the welfare of children or due to the fact that divorce may affect their social standing and career. It is sometimes easier to live with an unsatisfactory marriage than to face public comments.

But what constitutes a successful marriage? It includes both partners living together discussing their problems, understanding one another and willingly sharing their marital roles.

Marriage can be broadly divided in 3 phases.

- Initial five years of marriage during which the breakdown is the result of the failure to establish the necessary minimal physical and emotional relationship.
- Second phase of family life involving children, non employed wife, parents and changing needs of the family.
- Third phase after 25 years of marriage after the children have left home for their jobs and the housewife is coping with menopausal syndrome.

Childless marriages are more prone to divorce.

Only money cannot bring happiness in marriage. Excess of easy money provides opportunities to move in higher circles, attending late night parties and involving in extramarital sex.

Lack of money also does not meet your daily requirements creating cracks in the family bond. Mother in law may remain unsatisfied if the daughter in law is not from a rich family.

One should remember that most of women will respond with loyalty and affection if their husbands display consideration and interest in them, instead of taking them for granted.

Where the communication goes wrong in a relationship every thing seems to create a problem. A reminder by the partner will be misunderstood as nagging. Questions will be taken as provocations.

A man should understand that woman by nature will not like to be undermined by comparison to some other woman. A blue eyed wife whose husband always admires black eyes is bound to feel hurt. Wife with a short hair cut will not like her husband appreciating long thick hair.

In modern society sexual disharmony may be a source of conflict. Fulfilling sex involves closeness, caring and sharing. Such couples know how to touch each other. They realise that hand holding, hugging & kissing communicates love better and keeps erotic feelings simmering.

They keep the romance alive by remembering birthdays, anniversaries and giving presents to each other. They keep their sexual anticipation alive. By taking initiative one can break the deadlock or impasse.

Even if your husband is not behaving in the desired fashion

you should not be cold and indifferent towards him. Try to understand his problem which he may be facing in office or otherwise. Most couples should know how and when to say 'I love you' and 'sorry'.

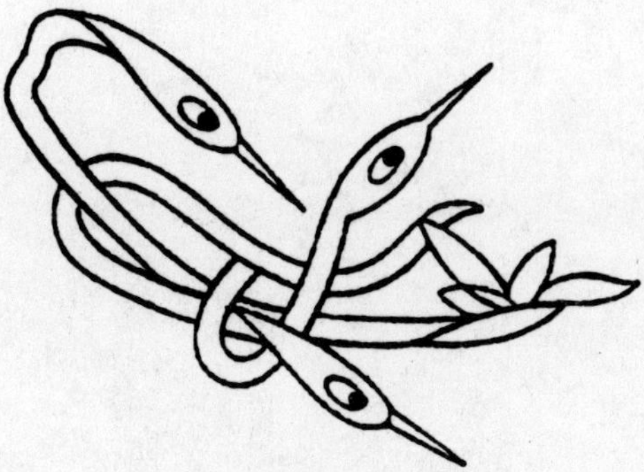

MARITAL COMPATIBILITY ACCORDING TO SUN SIGNS

In Hindus before marriage pandits are consulted to know whether the marriage will be a successful one or not studying their time and date of birth and sun signs. Here we are discussing by different combinations.

Aries - Aries

These people attract each other with sparks of passion and a lot of vitality.

- Aries - Taurus

It may not be a successful match. Taurus must come out of its ruts and Aries should become more practical.

- Aries - Gemini

Aries are emotional while Gemini believes on their mind. This may be a hot passionate couple.

- Aries - Cancer

Aries is like fire and cancer like water. The result may be steam so an intimate relationship will be difficult. Aries is the out going type while Cancer wants to remain in the house.

- Aries - Leo

These two fire signs can create a positive blaze. Both are egoistic yet the relationship can succeed at all levels of love and marriage.

- Aries - Virgo

There is little mutual ground between the two. This can be a tricky relationship.

- Aries - Libra

Libra is gentle, sensitive and romantic. This will be a good relationship.

- Aries - Scorpio

Scorpio is more sexy and aggressive. There will be a successful love affair culminating in marriage.

- Aries - Sagittarius

It will be an ideal marriage. There will be a natural give and take in the relationship. Excellent one in love, sex in pleasure.

- Aries - Capricorn

In this marriage Aries has to adjust to the Capricorn's ego.

- Aries - Aquarius

It is a relationship of fun. Marriage may finish up as a complicated game, because Aquarius is erratic and ecentric.

- Aries - Pisces

Marriage requires a delicate approach. There may be some emotional turmoil.

Taurus - Taurus

Both like physical, material and emotional comforts. They may be good friends instead of a husband and wife.

- Taurus - Gemini

A Gemini loves freedom while aTaurean is known for sensuality and a deep seated need to own and to hold things. It is a relationship to be entered into at one's own peril.

- Taurus - Cancer

This will prove to be a very good relationship although they will criticize each other occasionally.

- Taurus - Leo

Both like good food, luxury and the best things, in life, but both are adamant to do things in their own way. This may result in a difficult relationship.

- Taurus - Virgo

Mutual outlook on life makes it an exemplary partnership. Virgo is attracted to the Taurus elegance.

- Taurus - Libra

Both have interest in art, good food and conversation. Both signs are ruled by Venus so there will be a successful love affair. Libra is in the habit of changing love objects.

- Taurus - Scorpio

There may be an attraction of the opposite sex. Taurus is ruled by common sense while Scorpio uses its intuition and deep emotions. There may not be a long term relationship.

- Taurus - Sagittarius

In marriage there will persist a long term frustration.

- Taurus - Capricorn

Both have common objectives and will have an admirable relationship.

- Taurus - Aquarius

This will make for a short lived affair. Aquarius is the least conventional lover.

- Taurus - Pisces

This is not a successful alliance. A Piscean is sentimental and artistic while Taurus brings in a feeling of being wanted and needed.

Gemini - Gemini

There will be two physical bodies in this combination. It can be a compatible partnership but exhausting.

- Gemini - Cancer

There will be a difficult relationship.

- Gemini - Leo

In the long run it is doubtful that either one can cope.

- Gemini - Virgo

It will make for an unpredictable relationship. Both can be good friends and can analyse themselves and others instead of entering a several relationship.

- Gemini - Libra

This combination will make a relationship of happiness with better understanding.

- Gemini - Scorpio

Gemini enjoys passionate sexual demands otherwise these are likely to tear each other resulting in an unwise relationship.

- Gemini - Sagittarius

There will be a superficial relationship. Both parties may be involved in multiple relationships.

- Gemini - Capricorn

This is not an ideal match because none will change to meet the requirement of the other.

- Gemini - Aquarius

It will make an excellent relationship.

- Gemini - Pisces

Pisces is intuitive, adaptable and romantic while Gemini may indulge in drinking.

Cancer - Cancer

Both can bring each other's romantic and sexual dreams come true. Both are sensitive and will make an excellent relationship.

- Cancer - Leo

It will make for an unwise relationship.

- Cancer - Virgo

Virgo will hardly cope up with the needs of a cancerian.

- Cancer - Libra

Not a wise union. Cancer will be battering the relationship.

- Cancer - Sagittarius

Fire and water type relationship. There will be constant quarrelling upto the finish.

- Cancer - Capricorn

These are two opposites and will be financial wizards. But the Relationship does have hope.

- Cancer - Aquarius

Both are diverse personalities and will not be able to compromise.

- Cancer - Pisces

It will make an excellent match. Attraction will be instantaneous.

Leo - Leo

This is a pretty exotic coupling and will prove to be a difficult relationship.

- Leo - Virgo

Leo's need for constant attention brings boredom to Virgo after a while and in the long run will make an unwise relationship.

- Leo - Libra

Both share a love of luxury and flattery. A good relationship for a sexual affair.

- Leo - Scorpio

There will be a love hate relationship. Marriage will be most unwise.

- Leo - Sagittarius

Both are fire signs so they are half way to success even before they begin.

- Leo - Capricorn

A Leo finds, it difficult to understand a Capricorn. Relationship is best confined to the office only.

- Leo - Aquarius

If these do manage to get together then this can be an excellent combination of talents but unlikely for a long duration.

- Leo - Pisces

They denote Fire and water and hence a difficult combination.

Virgo - Virgo

Two virgos have a lot in common but a relationship is unlikely to work as they are likely to heap criticism upon each other.

- Virgo - Libra

Libra likes to spend money on things which the Virgo considers unnecessary. This is an unlikely union.

- Virgo - Scorpio

Relation is based on sexual attraction so long as two critics leave their sharp minds out side the bed room door. Good for business partnership only.

- Virgo - Sagittarius

Sagittarius usually wants a friend as well as a lover but a Virgo is not able to tolerate spontaneity. It will not make a satisfactory relationship.

- Virgo - Capricorn

They will make a good, happy love life. They will love each other in making an excellent union.

- Virgo - Aquarius

It is difficult to imagine these two together. An Aquarian may bring too much confusion.

- Virgo - Pisces

It will make a good partnership in business only.

Libra - Libra

Two Librans in harness make a perfect combination but chances are there that one may have an extra marital flirtation.

- Libra - Scorpio

Scorpio is notoriously jealous of the libra's roving eye, so in the long run there may be disastrous results.

- Libra - Sagittarius

Libra is attracted to him. An ideal relationship if based on friendship.

- Libra - Capricorn

Capricorn provide the stability that Libra desperately desires. An okay partners.

- Libra - Aquarius

It is a relationship which can work at all levels. Each understand, the need of the other.

- Libra - Pisces

There will be tremendous amount of affection and romance between two, but may not last for ever.

Scorpio - Scorpio

Both partners are unsure of themselves and therefore jealous. A Lengthy relationship our be a difficult task, nerve shattering and exhausting.

- Scorpio - Sagittarius

They should forget it as the combination will not work.

- Scorpio - Capricorn

Scorpio is forceful and powerful while a Capricorn is single minded. There will always be a clash.

- Scorpio - Aquarius

Too much of a compromise is needed for two to make a lasting relationship.

- Scorpio - Pisces

Both are very possessive, if both decide to possess each other they may log in for life.

Sagittarius - Sagittarius

This combination usually does not work. Odd enough. A Sense of freedom will be missing.

- Sagittarius - Aquarius

Aquarian will help the sagittarian to grow and expand to make a perfect relationship.

- Sagittarius - Pisces

The couple will be very heavy going. One is heartless and hardly promising for any relationship.

- Capricorn - Capricorn

Relationship will not survive.

- Capricorn - Aquarius

Intellectually these two possess tremendous insight and incisiveness which are bound to bring them together. But the two will find it hard to compromise.

- Capricorn - Pisces

Dependant Pisces loves Capricorn dominance. Capricorn thinks Piscean intution immensely useful. Partnership may succeed.

Aquarius - Aquarius

Sexual attraction is strong between them and both are equally ready to experiment. In other spheres they have to learn to respect the feelings of others.

Aquarius - Pisces

Piscean can go on giving and in the last may lose patience. It will be a one sided affair.

Pisces - Pisces

This affectionate and loving relationship can be nearly perfect. Both like beauty, peace and life at home.

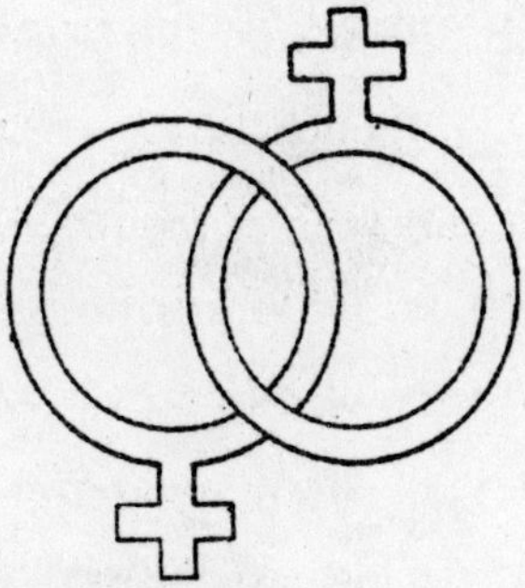

Rainbow of Life

Blue is the colour which makes you think,
White is the colour which likes to blink,
Red is the colour which shines to bright,
Black is the colour which scares you at night,

Purple is the colour which is so cute,
Green is the colour which plays the flute,
Pink is the colour which is sweeter than sugar
Grey is the colour which makes you to hit trigger

These are your colours of love, rainbow of life
Home can be made heaven by devoted wife.

–PRIYAM KOTWAL

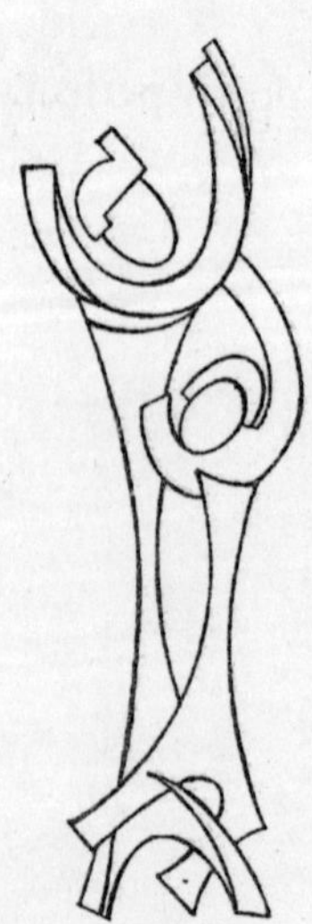

Intellectually these two possess tremendous insight and incisiveness which are bound to bring them together. But the two will find it hard to compromise.

- Capricorn - Pisces

Dependant Pisces loves Capricorn dominance. Capricorn thinks Piscean intution immensely useful. Partnership may succeed.

Aquarius - Aquarius

Sexual attraction is strong between them and both are equally ready to experiment. In other spheres they have to learn to respect the feelings of others.

Aquarius - Pisces

Piscean can go on giving and in the last may lose patience. It will be a one sided affair.

Pisces - Pisces

This affectionate and loving relationship can be nearly perfect. Both like beauty, peace and life at home.

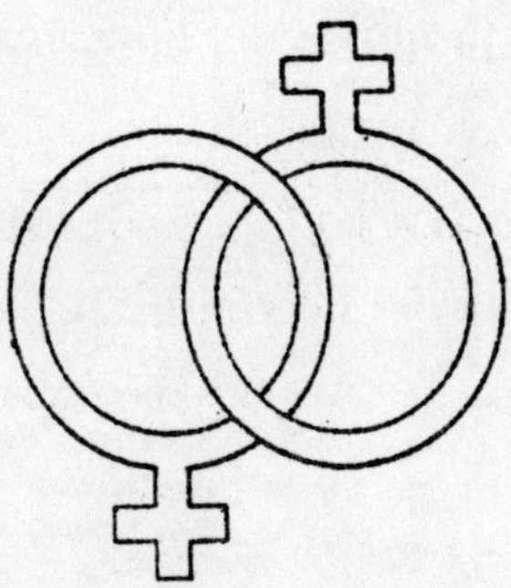

Rainbow of Life

Blue is the colour which makes you think,
White is the colour which likes to blink,
Red is the colour which shines to bright,
Black is the colour which scares you at night,

Purple is the colour which is so cute,
Green is the colour which plays the flute,
Pink is the colour which is sweeter than sugar
Grey is the colour which makes you to hit trigger

These are your colours of love, rainbow of life
Home can be made heaven by devoted wife.

–PRIYAM KOTWAL

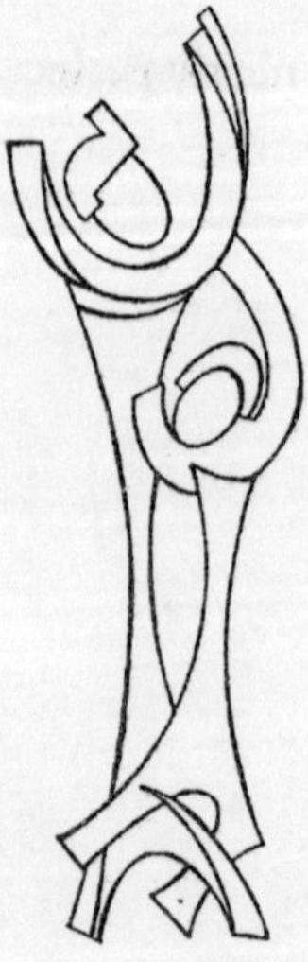